"This reads like an informative and enjoyable clinical conversation, providing a comprehensive knowledge base through accessible explanations of the theory behind voice therapy, its practical application, and links to pertinent research literature. Self-development activities enable reflective practice for voice patients and beyond! Clinical tips offer a systematic way to build knowledge or provide a "go-to" resource for a focused approach. This is set to be a valued clinical companion."
Fiona Williams, Band 5 / Newly Qualified Speech and Language Therapist

"As a newly qualified practitioner, a strong clinical resource provides not only advice but a sense of reassurance. This book does exactly that – clear & concise, it provides a supportive easy to read guide for navigating the world of voice disorders."
Saba Jennings, Band 6 Community Speech and Language Therapist

ACCESS YOUR ONLINE RESOURCES

Navigating Voice Disorders is accompanied by a number of printable online materials, designed to ensure this resource best supports your professional needs.

Activate your online resources:

Go to www.routledge.com/cw/speechmark and click on the cover of this book.

Click the "Sign in or Request Access" button and follow the instructions in order to access the resources.

NAVIGATING VOICE DISORDERS

This book comprises 50 tips for speech and language therapy practitioners who are new to, or less experienced in, working with adult voice disorders. It considers the full clinical pathway from assessment to management and on through to discharge.

Packed with easily accessible, practical hints about therapy and useful self-development activities for the reader, sections cover:

- Reflecting on the normal voice
- 'Doing' therapy
- Assessment
- Management
- Specific diagnoses
- Professional voice users
- Professional liason
- Learning from clients

The resource concludes with a handy appendix providing further reading and useful resources. Presenting diagnosis-specific and client group-specific tips alongside widely applicable guidance, this is a go-to book for accessible and practical support for voice newbies.

Carolyn Andrews is a speech and language therapist and University Teaching Fellow with over 20 years' clinical experience and education of SLT students. She first got curious about the voice by listening to Top of the Pops in the 1980s and is fascinated by the uniqueness of our voices. Carolyn sees a key part of professional practice as translating complicated theory into accessible knowledge for clients and students alike, and loves exploring the craft of the voice with others.

NAVIGATING SPEECH AND LANGUAGE THERAPY

Navigating the field of speech and language therapy can seem overwhelming to students and newly qualified therapists. This series is designed to provide concise, entry-level summaries of key areas in speech and language therapy, providing a basic insight into a specific area of therapy. Comprising practical advice and guidance from an expert in the field, the books cover topics such as assessment, therapy, psychological approaches, and onward referral. This is a useful tool for anyone new to speech and language therapy, or building confidence in their field.

Navigating Adult Stammering
100 Points for Speech and Language Therapists
Trudy Stewart

Navigating Telehealth for Speech and Language Therapists
The Remotely Possible in 50 Key Points
Rebekah Davies

Navigating AAC
50 Essential Strategies and Resources for Using Augmentative and Alternative Communication
Alison Battye

Navigating Voice Disorders
Around the Larynx in 50 Tips
Carolyn Andrews

NAVIGATING VOICE DISORDERS

AROUND THE LARYNX IN 50 TIPS

Carolyn Andrews

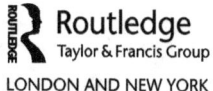

LONDON AND NEW YORK

Cover image: © Getty Images

First published 2023
by Routledge
4 Park Square, Milton Park, Abingdon, Oxon OX14 4RN

and by Routledge
605 Third Avenue, New York, NY 10158

Routledge is an imprint of the Taylor & Francis Group, an informa business

© 2023 Carolyn Andrews

The right of Carolyn Andrews to be identified as author of this work has been asserted in accordance with sections 77 and 78 of the Copyright, Designs and Patents Act 1988.

All rights reserved. The purchase of this copyright material confers the right on the purchasing institution to photocopy or download pages which bear the companion website and a copyright line at the bottom of the page. No other parts of this book may be reprinted or reproduced or utilised in any form or by any electronic, mechanical, or other means, now known or hereafter invented, including photocopying and recording, or in any information storage or retrieval system, without permission in writing from the publishers.

Trademark notice: Product or corporate names may be trademarks or registered trademarks, and are used only for identification and explanation without intent to infringe.

British Library Cataloguing-in-Publication Data
A catalogue record for this book is available from the British Library

Library of Congress Cataloging-in-Publication Data
Names: Andrews, Carolyn, (Speech and language therapist), author.
Title: Navigating voice disorders : around the larynx in 50 tips / Carolyn Andrews.
Description: First edition. | Abingdon, Oxon ; New York, NY : Routledge, 2023. |
Series: Navigating speech and language therapy ; 4 |
Includes bibliographical references and index. |
Identifiers: LCCN 2022025565 (print) | LCCN 2022025566 (ebook) |
ISBN 9781032157290 (pbk) | ISBN 9781032157276 (hbk) |
ISBN 9781003245452 (ebk)
Subjects: LCSH: Voice disorders. | Speech disorders.
Classification: LCC RF510 .A49 2023 (print) |
LCC RF510 (ebook) | DDC 616.85/56–dc23/eng/20220913
LC record available at https://lccn.loc.gov/2022025565
LC ebook record available at https://lccn.loc.gov/2022025566

ISBN: 978-1-032-15727-6 (hbk)
ISBN: 978-1-032-15729-0 (pbk)
ISBN: 978-1-003-24545-2 (ebk)

DOI: 10.4324/9781003245452

Typeset in Aldus
by Newgen Publishing UK

Access the companion website: www.routledge.com/cw/speechmark

CONTENTS

List of figures	x
Acknowledgements	xi

Chapter 1
INTRODUCTION   1

Chapter 2
YOUR VOICE, THE NORMAL VOICE   12

Tip 1 – How's *your* voice?	13
Tip 2 – Be your own client	15
Tip 3 – The world is your voice clinic!	18

Chapter 3
"DOING" VOICE THERAPY   21

Tip 4 – Understanding change	22
Tip 5 – Working collaboratively	27
Tip 6 – The client as active agent	29
Tip 7 – Cultivating tender conversations	32
Tip 8 – Remote vs. face-to-face therapy	36
Tip 9 – A blend of SLT personalities	39
Tip 10 – Giving feedback	43
Tip 11 – Defining outcomes	46
Tip 12 – When progress slows	51
Tip 13 – Being a culturally responsive therapist	55

Chapter 4
ASSESSMENT   62

Tip 14 – An assessment checklist	63
Tip 15 – Judging amount of voice use	69

Tip 16 – Assessment as experimentation 72
Tip 17 – Summarising your findings: what's in a label? 74
Tip 18 – To plan therapy or not? 78

Chapter 5
MANAGEMENT 86

Tip 19 – Creating a therapy plan 87
Tip 20 – Indirect therapy 91
Tip 21 – Nurturing a healthy mind–body connection 96
Tip 22 – Awareness, awareness, awareness! 98
Tip 23 – Hear it, feel it, locate it 102
Tip 24 – Just breathe… 104
Tip 25 – Semi-occluded vocal tract therapy 109
Tip 26 – Break it down or build it up? 114

Chapter 6
WORKING WITH SPECIFIC DIAGNOSES 122

Tip 27 – Functional voice disorder 123
Tip 28 – Psychogenic voice disorder 129
Tip 29 – Vocal fold nodules 132
Tip 30 – Reinke's oedema 138
Tip 31 – Granulomas 141
Tip 32 – Vocal fold palsies 143
Tip 33 – Upper airway disorders 148
Tip 34 – Presbyphonia 151
Tip 35 – Spasmodic dysphonia 154
Tip 36 – Preparing for surgery 156
Tip 37 – Laryngeal papilloma 160
Tip 38 – Vocal fold polyps 163
Tip 39 – Vocal fold cysts 164

Chapter 7
WORKING WITH PROFESSIONAL VOICE USERS 172

Tip 40 – Vocal athletes 173
Tip 41 – Educators 176

Tip 42 – Contact centre workers 182
Tip 43 – Clients in the arts industry 185
Tip 44 – Clients in the fitness industry 190
Tip 45 – Vocal warm-ups and cool-downs 192

Chapter 8
PROFESSIONAL LIAISON 198

Tip 46 – Support for ... physical health 199
Tip 47 – Support for ... mental health 202
Tip 48 – Support for ... smoking cessation 204
Tip 49 – Support for ... employment 206
Tip 50 – Multidisciplinary work in action 208

Chapter 9
LEARNING FROM CLIENTS 211

Learn from ... Amanda Lynne 212
Learn from ... Rory 214
Learn from ... Eliza Kath 218

Appendix 1: Published assessments 220
Appendix 2: Therapy resources 224
Useful resources 227
Index 229

FIGURES

1	Summary of helpers and hindrances to behavioural change	25
2	The social-cognitive concepts contributing to client responsibility for practice	29
3	The different roles of a speech and language therapist	39
4	The potential wider community positively impacted by SLT input	49
5	Classification of voice disorders	75
6	Sample summary of the 4P influencing factors for a client	77
7	The cycle of throat clearing and irritation	93
8a	A more difficult voice weighs more heavily before therapy	117
8b	More equally weighted use of effective and less effective voice use	118
8c	Effective voice outweighs ineffective voice use	118
9	The cumulative effect of tension with the voice	125
10a	Normal vocal fold position at rest and on phonation	144
10b	Impact of a left abducted VFP at rest and on phonation	144
10c	Impact of a left adducted VFP at rest and on phonation	145
11	The three stages of SLT intervention for surgical voice clients	156
12	A cycle of SLT input in relation to papilloma growth	161

ACKNOWLEDGEMENTS

This book would not have been possible without the support of family, friends, and colleagues. Many thanks go to:

My family for their encouragement, belief, and for their interest in the magical world of voice even when fun vocal facts had not been solicited!

Valerie Campbell, SLT colleague and valued friend, who employed me as a newly qualified therapist and believed in her team to shape the therapist I am today.

Fiona MacGregor, my Ear, Nose and Throat Consultant colleague, whose joint Voice Clinic and passion about the voice nurtured my own growth in the field and led to our fruitful collaboration

My fellow voice geeks, Rose, Sarah, Kirsty, and Stephen, for their own insights as therapists which confirmed my early ideas for this book.

The clients who shared their experiences of voice therapy so you can understand therapy-in-action.

Chapter 1

INTRODUCTION

The voice is fascinating! In this chapter I introduce what it means to have a voice and the impact of not having a voice for the speaker, listeners, and the wider economy. I outline the clinical wisdom you can expect from the rest of the book and where to head to develop your understanding of voice-related topics beyond the scope of this resource. You'll learn about my non-linear entry to voicework and, I hope, be inspired by the life-changing impact you can have on a client's life.

WHAT DOES IT MEAN TO HAVE A VOICE?

To have a voice has two meanings. Firstly, and in layperson's terms, it means we're capable of producing noise from our larynx, or voice box (the source) which is shaped by other structures in our vocal tract (the filter) to produce verbal communication. Secondly, having a voice means we have the freedom to share thoughts and opinions, verbally or through alternative means of communication.

What, then, does not having a voice mean? For some, being marginalised through a stigmatised condition (such as autism or stammering) or oppressed personal characteristic (such as religious affiliation, skin colour, sexuality, gender identity, or political connection) leaves the speaker feeling unheard. At a professional level the Royal College of Speech and Language Therapists is committed to ensuring UK members' and service users' voices are heard, and you and I can work to ensure individual clients' experiences are also promoted. Alternatively, not having a voice equates with temporary or permanent change to the speaker's voice quality and a relative or friend might say "I've lost my voice", referring to any change from no phonation at all to mild hoarseness.

As speech and language therapists (SLTs), we want our clients to have a voice in both senses of the term but this book focuses on the latter interpretation of voicework.

THE IMPACT OF NOT HAVING A VOICE

In taking our voices for granted, we may only notice them when they don't work but, unlike hips or knees, they can't be replaced. Normal voices don't often make the news headlines but failing or difficult voices *do*, particularly when the speaker is in the public eye. In 2017, a British politician's persistent cough and vocal strain at her political party's conference was covered by major news outlets and in an interview in 2018, it was brought up again. Publicly observed voice difficulties are not easily forgotten! High-profile singers including Adele, Sam Smith, Jessie J, Jess Glynn, and James Blunt have all acknowledged problematic singing voices which have even made their way to Hollywood where vocal fold nodules were used as inaccurate drama in the first of the Pitch Perfect films.

Regardless of the aetiology, and regardless of whether the speaker holds a high-profile position, any voice alteration can be upsetting and frustrating. Voices contribute to our identity – they are how we are recognised, how we make our presence known, sometimes how we are judged and even how we flirt (Hughes et al., 2010)! Voice problems can be hindering in the workplace (e.g. Van Houtte et al., 2011; Spellman, 2020) with psychological and financial consequences for the client and economic burden if replacement staff are required. They can compromise clients' perception of overall quality of life (e.g. Wilson et al., 2002; Mansouri et al., in press) and some clients consider moderate dysphonia to be comparable to monocular blindness (Naunheim et al., 2020).

For the listener, dysphonic voices may be perceived as less credible (Schroeder et al., 2020) or less intelligible (Porcaro et al., 2020) and can increase the listener's cognitive demand as they concentrate on what is being said (Evitts et al., 2016), particularly with background noise (Ishikawa et al., 2017). Alongside listener frustration, more serious consequences exist for teachers working with children who struggle to understand dysphonic instructions (Lyberg-Åhlander et al., 2015; Chiu & Ma, 2019) and for air traffic controllers responsible for the safety of passengers and crew (Villar et al., 2016; Korn et al., 2019). Inanimate listeners are not even spared the challenges – voice recognition systems for TV remote controls, telephone banking or home entertainment rely on clear voices and are less able to process dysphonia (Rohlfing et al., 2021). Sure enough, when I gave instructions to our Alexa™ using strained or breathy voice qualities, my musical requests were either ignored or met with "I can't find that song".

With impact reaching the speaker, the listener, and the economy, working with the disordered voice is important and valuable, and you'll soon discover that regardless of what originally brought your client to you, your support may change their life in ways you or they may never had anticipated. The short meditations you recommend to develop awareness of the breath and ease of tension in the mind (Tip 22) may become a regular routine which supports stress management. The explanation you give around the harm of smoking (Tip 48) may just be the nudge for clients to finally commit to stopping for the good of their wider health. And the active listening you've exuded while exploring the connection between stress and their voice (Tip 7) may facilitate a search for onward counselling support in relation to non-voice-related stressors (Tip 47). I've met performers who have considered a change of career upon reflection of their occupational voice demands. I've met teachers who have retired from teaching early after reflecting on the influence of work stress and I've met clients who have continued to work, having previously thought this wasn't possible with a vocal fold palsy or recurring laryngeal papillomas. Voice therapy can become part of overall life change and improved self-care, and as voice therapists we're in a privileged position to share that.

WHAT TO EXPECT FROM THIS BOOK

Fifty clinical tips which focus on key knowledge for your early voice adventures are complemented by 24 self-development activities which I strongly encourage you to try. These develop your clinical skills practice, comfort in your own voice experimentation, and help you to empathise with the possible challenges for clients in developing a new voice-related routine. Some of Rumbach et al.'s (2021) speech and language therapy (SLT) students were concerned that a lack of performance or singing background was disadvantageous to voicework but it isn't. I'm still exploring what my voice can do but that doesn't mean I'm an ineffective voice therapist! Instructions are provided with each self-development activity, and you can either make notes in the appendices or download the supporting template from www.routledge.com/cw/speechmark and file your thoughts in your personal development plan. You can start your learning with Tip 1 and work through each tip in turn, or you can search for the topics of particular relevance for your current clients, using the cross-referencing between tips to build your knowledge within a specific area of voicework.

Why these particular tips? Well, my choices have been influenced by: the research literature around student development in voice therapy (Iwarsson, 2015; Rumbach et al., 2021); my clinical experience and what I consider fundamental aspects of voicework; my reflections on supervising students and mentoring newly qualified therapists; and thoughts from SLT colleagues and students. However, these tips are not all you need to know, or can know, to work with the voice. I have written this book assuming you already have a grounding in core head and neck structures, cranial nerves and their functions, and the complexities of phonetics. If these subjects are a little rusty, I would return to your notes for some revision and access the following additional resources. Dimon (2018) is a useful refresher of voice anatomy and Brassett et al. (2017) provide a beautiful account of the origins of anatomy terms to help you remember the meaning of each. Did you know that thyroid means shield-shaped, like the thyroid cartilage, or pterygoid comes from the Latin for wing (pteryx) as the lateral pterygoid resembles a spread of feathers? Academic texts such as Mathieson (2013) and Sapienza and Hoffman (2022) provide theoretical knowledge, and clinical texts such as Shewell (2009) and Martin (2021) supply a wealth of therapeutic exercises. I also recommend you research the voice clinical guidelines produced by your relevant professional body – although there will be international overlap, you should ensure you are practicing within your own state or national guidance. Additionally, the literature peppered across the tips signposts you to further reading to develop your understanding and for interest.

This book focuses on adult voice difficulties. Although the vocal tract is not fully mature until the age of 20 (Mathieson, 2013), UK adult SLT services generally support clients from 18 years old, working with slightly younger clients if they've left school or are pursuing a performing arts career where early voicework is a wise investment in longer term vocal health. Voice changes associated with laryngeal cancer are beyond the scope of the book as they are influenced by radical surgical intervention and/or radiotherapy and I additionally do not discuss the transgender voice. Some skills used in relation to dysphonia will be relevant for developing a passing transgender voice but this is a topic all of its own so instead I direct you Adler (2019) as a theoretical text, and Christella Antoni, a leading clinician in the UK working with this population, has some useful video resources on her website.

VOICEWORK AND ME

Although I now have many years of voice experience, I wasn't born knowing what I know now. My earliest curiosity around the voice was watching Top of the Pops, a UK weekly music show, in the 1980s and 1990s. I remember mimicking different voice styles which ranged from the twang in Fine Young Cannibals' *She Drives Me Crazy* to the wide pitch ranges of Whitney Houston and A-Ha's Morten Harket (many of my male singing clients still refer to Morten's ability to reach high notes) and I was intrigued by the deep pitch of Leonard Cohen and Bonnie Tyler's huskiness which she later attributed to surgery for vocal fold nodules. More recent voices with distinctive qualities include Janice, a character from the sitcom *Friends*, and I wonder what voices have pricked up your ears?

Despite this early curiosity around the voice, my road to being a specialist voice therapist hasn't been direct. My supervising therapist during my final year adult voice placement was an excellent educator but I found myself longing for a stroke caseload with which I'd connected during my previous year of study. The exam on this final placement was a session watched live by a university lecturer but my client arrived with all problems now resolved which I hadn't been expecting – I'd assumed every difficulty required therapy! Around the same time I knew another therapist who smoked and a friend with nodules openly declared she wasn't going to follow SLT advice (more of that in Tip 29). All in all, I found it difficult to envision my role with voice clients. Fast forward more than 20 years and I'm fascinated by vocal changes which emerge from a small tweak of the vocal tract, and the whole-body approach is both scientifically and personally sound. Why am I telling you all of this? Well, I want you to see this book as a clinical friend, written from a place of understanding about the challenges with an adult voice caseload but equally from a place of passion for all things voice-related. I envisage that you might thumb through this on the bus to and from placement, or perhaps use it during personal development time in the early months of a new job or rotation in to voice.

Across the years I've had the pleasure of sharing curiosity about the voice with fabulous SLT and Ear, Nose, and Throat colleagues. We've asked questions of our own practice; we've collectively explored vocal wonders; and I hope you too can access direct support as you dive into this field. If you're a student, you'll have a supervising therapist on placement to support your clinical development and if you're a newly qualified or returning therapist, you may well have a more experienced clinician on hand. For some readers, your contact may be someone working academically. All these mentors can share their clinical expertise and provide feedback on your own voice skills so you know exactly what is meant by pitch glides, a resonant voice or anything else you're not sure of (Rumbach et al., 2021). Do use them to support your development!

TERMINOLOGY

Throughout the book "client" has been used over "patient" as a less pathologising term though many clients describe themselves as patients, influenced by societal and media use of the term. I recognise "client" implies services are being paid for and in the UK the National Health Service is free at the point of delivery, but I see this as a warmer term than "service user". "They", "them", and "their" replace gender-specific pronouns unless the evidence base relates to a specific gender, and speech and language therapist is used over speech and language pathologist as the book has been written in the UK, though these terms are interchangeable.

Finally, I often use the collective term of "we" as I want you to see this as a collaborative exploration of voice. Even if your next placement is with a different specialism, or you decide other clinical fields are your preferences, for now you are part of a dynamic community of professionals, passionate about the voice and the impact SLT can have for those experiencing difficulties. As you take your first steps on your voice adventures, know that you are about to make a real difference. Welcome to our world!

REFERENCES

Adler, R. K. (Ed.) (2019) *Voice and Communication therapy for the transgender/gender diverse client: a comprehensive guide* (3rd Ed). San Diego: Plural Publishing

Brassett, C., Evans, E. & Fay, I. (2017) *The Secret Language of Anatomy. An Illustrated Guide to the Origins of Anatomical Terms.* Chichester: Anatomy Boutique Books

Chiu, J, C-H. & Ma, E. P-M. (2019) The Impact of Dysphonic Voices on Children's Comprehension of Spoken Language. *Journal of Voice* 33 (5) 801.e7–801.e16 https://doi.org/10.1016/j.jvoice.2018.03.004

Dimon, T. (2018) *Anatomy of the Voice. An Illustrated Guide for Singers, Vocal Coaches, and Speech Therapists.* Berkeley: North Atlantic Books

Evitts, P.M., Starmer, H., Teets, K., Montgomery, C., Calhoun, L., Schulze, A., MacKenzie, J. & Adams, L. (2016) The impact of dysphonic voices on healthy listeners: Listener reaction times, speech intelligibility, and listener comprehension. *American Journal of Speech-Language Pathology* 25 (4) 561–575 https://dx.doi.org/10.1044/2016_AJSLP-14-0183

Hughes, S. M., Farley, S. D. & Rhodes, B. C. (2010) Vocal and Physiological Changes in Response to the Physical Attractiveness of Conversational Partners. *Journal of Nonverbal Behavior* 34 (3) 155–167 https://doi.org/10.1007/s10919-010-0087-9

Ishikawa, K. Boyce, S., Kelchner, L., Powell, M. G., Schieve, H., de Alarcon, A. & Khosla, S. (2017) The effect of background noise on intelligibility of dysphonic speech.

Journal of Speech, Language and Hearing Research 60 (7) 1919–1929 https://doi.org/10.1044/2017_JSLHR-S-16-0012

Iwarsson, J. (2015) Reflections on clinical expertise and silent know-how in voice therapy. *Logopedics Phoniatrics Vocology* 40 (2) 66–71 https://doi.org/10.3109/14015439.2014.949302

Korn, G. P., Villar, A. C. & Azevedo, R. R. (2019) Hoarseness and vocal tract discomfort and associated risk factors in air traffic controllers. *Brazilian Journal of Otorhinolaryngology* 85 (3) 329–336 https://doi.org/10.1016/j.bjorl.2018.02.009

Lyberg-Åhlander, V., Brännström, K. J. & Sahlén, B. S. (2015) On the interaction of speakers' voice quality, ambient noise and task complexity with children's listening comprehension and cognition. *Frontiers in Psychology* 6 https://doi.org/10.3389/fpsyg.2015.00871

Mansouri, Y., Naderifar, E., Hajiyakchali, A. & Moradi, N. (in press) The Relationship Between Dysphonia Severity Index and Voice-Related Quality of Life in the Elementary School Teachers with Voice Complaint. *Journal of Voice* https://doi.org/10.1016/j.jvoice.2021.02.017

Martin, S. (2021) *Working With Voice Disorders. Theory and Practice.* (3rd Ed.) Abingdon: Routledge

Mathieson, L. (2013) *Greene and Mathieson's The Voice and its Disorders* (6th Ed.) Hoboken: Wiley

Naunheim, M. R., Goldberg, L., Bai, J. B., Rubinstein, B. J. & Courey, M. S. (2020) Measuring the Impact of Dysphonia on Quality of Life Using Health State Preferences. *The Laryngoscope* 130 (4) E177-E182 https://doi.org/10.1002/lary.28148

Porcaro, C. K., Evitts, P. M., King, N., Hood, C., Campbell, E., White, L. & Veraguas, J. (2020) Effect of Dysphonia and Cognitive-Perceptual Listener Strategies on Speech Intelligibility. *Journal of Voice* 34 (5) 806.e7–806.e18 https://doi.org/10.1016/j.jvoice.2019.03.013

Rohlfing, M. L., Buckley, D. P., Piraquive, J., Stepp, C. E. & Tracy, L. F. (2021) Hey Siri: How Effective are Common

Voice Recognition Systems at Recognizing Dysphonic Voice? *Laryngoscope 131* (7) 1599–1607 https://doi.org/10.1002/lary.29082

Rumbach, A. F., Dallaston, K. & Hill, A. E. (2021) Student perceptions of factors that influence clinical competency in voice. *International Journal of Speech-Language Pathology* 23 (2) https://doi.org/10.1080/17549507.2020.1737733

Sapienza, C. & Hoffman, B. (2022) *Voice disorders* (4th Ed.) San Diego: Plural Publishing

Schroeder, S. R., Rembrandt, H. N., May, S. &Freeman, M. R. (2020) Does having a voice disorder hurt credibility? *Journal of Communication Disorders 87* 106035 https://doi.org/j.jcomdis.2020.106035

Shewell, C. (2009) *Voice Work. Art and Science in Changing Voices*. Chichester: Wiley-Blackwell

Spellman, J., Coulter, M., Roth, C. & Johnson, C. (2020) Prevalence, Characteristics and Impact of Dysphonia in US Marine Corps Drill Instructors. *Journal of Voice 34* (5) 694–701 https://doi.org/10.1016/j.jvoice.2019.02.015

Van Houtte, E., Claeys, S., Wuyts, F. & Van Lierde, K. (2011) The Impact of Voice Disorders Among Teachers: Vocal Complaints, Treatment-Seeking Behaviour, Knowledge of Vocal Care, and Voice-Related Absenteeism. *Journal of Voice* 25 (5) 570–575 https://doi.org/10.1016/j.jvoice.2010.04.008

Villar, A. C. N. W. B., Korn, G. P. & Azevedo, R. R. (2016) Perceptual-auditory and Acoustic Analysis of Air Traffic Controllers' Voices Pre- and Postshift. *Journal of Voice* 30 (6) 768.e11–768.e15 https://doi.org/10.1016/j.jvoice.2015.10.021

Wilson, J. A. Deary, I. J., Millar, A. & MacKenzie, K. (2002) The quality of life impact of dysphonia. *Clinical Otolaryngology* 27 (3) 179–182 http://doi.org/10.1046/j.1365-2273.2002.00559.x

ADDITIONAL LEARNING RESOURCES

Voice Science Works – a website distilling contemporary research for use by any voice user. It has useful downloadable resources and educational videos. www.voicescienceworks.org/

SUGGESTED INSTAGRAM ACCOUNTS TO FOLLOW

@voicefituk – a UK specialist voice therapist, Tor Spence, runs this account. She has a particular interest in chronic cough and upper airway disorders

@voicecarecentre – a London voice centre specialising in vocal manual therapy. Their multidisciplinary team includes SLTs, a vocal rehab coach, an osteopath, a mindset coach, and nutritional scientist

@vocologyireland – a singing teacher, Eimar McCarthy Luddy, runs this account. She has an interest in vocal health for singing and loves her anatomy with fun quizzes and helpful diagrams to help the layperson understand the layout of the vocal tract

@kristie_voice – this is Kirstie Knickerbocker's account and I cite some of her work later. She is an American speech and language therapist and voice specialist

Chapter 2

YOUR VOICE, THE NORMAL VOICE

Most of this book considers the disordered voice, but paying attention to our experience of, and relationship with, a non-problematic voice gives a useful context for learning about dysphonia, and you can do this through reflection on *your* voice use and care. In this chapter your first three tips encourage you to use your own habits to step into clients' shoes and appreciate what voice therapy might mean for them. The everyday world can be your secret voice clinic and by listening to the spoken and sung voices around you, you can hone your observational and listening skills. Reflection is a key part of our development as practitioners and is often best done with no distractions, so find a space and half an hour to think about *you* as you work through this chapter. We'll soon come on to thinking about your clients!

TIP 1 – HOW'S *YOUR* VOICE?

Preparing to work with others' voices comes with an advantage – we all have one of our own! If we are to encourage others to change their voice care we should practice what we preach, and if we wish clients to experiment with voice exercises we should also consider how we connect with them ourselves. Such reflection guides us to be more empathetic and helps identify knowledge gaps or worries about our practice. Once we acknowledge missing theory or concerns, we can then take action to address them.

This tip considers your opinion of your voice, and how you have been looking after it up to now. It sets the scene for Tip 2 which highlights potential voice hazards in SLT and introduces our first voice experiments.

> **SELF-DEVELOPMENT ACTIVITY 1 – YOUR RELATIONSHIP WITH YOUR SPEAKING VOICE**
>
> Take a moment to think about the questions below – your reflections could consider your voice quality, pitch, volume, or the rate of your speech, as well as your confidence in allowing your voice to be heard. If there are other elements of your voice which spring to mind, include those too.
>
> - What do you like about your speaking voice?
> - Is there anything you would like to change about your speaking voice?
> - How does your voice reflect your identity?

Now let's think about your relationship with your singing voice which may be different from the connection with your speaking voice. I know mine is! As a teenager, I was told by a very musically talented friend that I couldn't sing and, believing their background to add credibility to this statement, I held it to be true for a long time and am still working to fully let go of it. This impacts on what I sing, where I sing, with whom I sing, and how much I belt out a song.

> **SELF-DEVELOPMENT ACTIVITY 2 – YOUR RELATIONSHIP WITH YOUR SINGING VOICE**
>
> - What do you like about your singing voice?
> - Is there anything you would like to change about your singing voice?
> - Are these changes related to technical aspects of singing, your self-confidence, or both?

Finally, let's consider your experience of vocal changes.

> **SELF-DEVELOPMENT ACTIVITY 3**
>
> - Have you ever experienced change(s) to your voice quality or even total voice loss?
> - What were the circumstances that led to this? How long did the change(s) last?
> - What were the consequences for you? Did they matter?
> - What action did you take in response to the voice changes?
> - If you were to experience similar change(s) now, would the consequence(s) be the same or would the impact be different from your previous experience(s)?

TIP 2 – BE YOUR OWN CLIENT

In the previous tip you reflected on your connection with your voice – now let's consider how you look after your voice because, just like the professional voice user groups in Chapter 7, we also rely on our voices as a tool of our trade. SLTs are not immune to difficulties and may experience vocal fatigue from long periods of speaking, speaking loudly, throat clearing, not drinking enough water, working in environments with background noise or air-conditioning, and problems from the way the voice is used outside of work (Joseph et al., 2020). Knickerbocker et al. (2021) further recognise that our voices may be challenged by the complexity of our communication, the wide range of people we communicate with, and the social and emotional aspects of our communication. Such hazards can subsequently lead to feelings of dryness in the throat, a tightness in the upper body, a sensation of choking, throat pain, and effortful speaking (Joseph et al., 2020) – everything our clients may report!

Research also highlights the difficulties SLT students experience (Gottliebson et al., 2007; van Lierde et al., 2010; Warhurst et al., 2012; Searl & Dargin, 2021). Interestingly, Searl and Dargin's (2021) student participants *overestimated* speaking time, water intake, and daily stress, and *underestimated* singing, second-hand smoke exposure, hours of sleep, caffeine intake, and alcohol intake. As you reflect on your own voice care, think comprehensively and holistically, taking heed that even professionals trained in voice are not exempt from problems. This all means we need to practice healthy voice care, whatever caseload we're working with. Even if your next placement or rotation is with a different caseload, do keep looking after your voice.

Occasionally clients ask if I follow my own advice and I acknowledge that I drink plenty of water, particularly when I am teaching. I use steam inhalations when I have a heavy day of voice use ahead or when I have a cold, and am attentive to the impact of awkward postures or stress, using head and neck stretches to relieve creeping tension. Rumbach et al.'s (2021)

SLT students recognised that if clinicians didn't look after their voices, it could be difficult to instil good voice care in others. A client is unlikely to stop throat clearing if you are doing this all the way through your session!

> ### SELF-DEVELOPMENT ACTIVITY 4 – BRINGING TOGETHER YOUR REFLECTIONS
>
> Combining your reflections from the previous tip with the research about SLTs and SLT students, what are your thoughts on your voice use and care?
>
> - What patterns are emerging with how you do, or do not, look after your voice on a day-to-day basis?
> - What patterns are emerging with how you do, or do not, look after your voice when it is struggling?
> - How does the quality of your care and use of your voice reflect the relationship you have with your voice?
> - What action could you take forward from these reflections?

As well as acting on your reflections above, try the next couple of self-development activities to develop your voice care.

> ### SELF-DEVELOPMENT ACTIVITY 5 – EXPERIMENTING WITH VOICE CONSERVATION
>
> Some clients benefit from voice rest as part of vocal healing but it's not always easy to resist the urge to speak. To understand the challenges associated with this guidance, let's try some voice conservation ourselves. Pick a day you usually have frequent conversations and try to have four hours of continuous voice rest. For the

purposes of the experiment, *when* you do this during the day doesn't matter as much as *how long* you do this.

- What challenges were there in not speaking to other people?
- Did you find yourself speaking before you realised?
- How did you prevent or respond to the challenges?
- Was there anything you weren't able to do because you were resting your voice?
- How did it feel to be silent?
- How did it feel to be instructed to be silent?

Self-development activity 6 – steam inhalations

Steam inhalations hydrate the vocal folds superficially and help to break up excessive secretions in the vocal tract. The added benefit is that sitting down to complete the inhalations and just breathing can be a real antidote to an otherwise busy day.

Using a bowl of water hot enough to emit steam, lean over the bowl with a towel over your head to retain the steam. You shouldn't use any menthol or eucalyptus oils as you're not using the steam to clear a cold – you're using it for superficial hydration. Breathe in the hot air for 10–15 minutes and then have 45 minutes' voice rest afterwards to allow dilated blood vessels to settle.

- What was this experience like?
- What was it like to sit and breathe without any opportunity to do anything else?
- How easy or difficult was it to incorporate the voice rest afterwards?

TIP 3 – THE WORLD IS YOUR VOICE CLINIC!

Every day and everywhere we are surrounded by different voices, some of which we find appealing and some we judge as irritating, though we need to be careful that voice preferences don't become unintended linguistic racism where judgements are made about education, status, or personality based on accents or dialectal form of language use.

Setting aside our vocal preferences, when all component parts work effectively and safely, *every* voice is a good voice and we can use the voices around us to extend our auditory-perceptual skills and awareness of different voice qualities (Rumbach et al., 2021). Your next self-development activity views the everyday world as your own voice clinic in which you can rate voices in the supermarket, on the bus, in a restaurant, in the university library, at home … anywhere really! If you attach a preferential judgement to your evaluation, notice this too, for awareness of your own prejudices will help you suspend these in clinical practice.

> **SELF-DEVELOPMENT ACTIVITY 7 – RATING OTHERS' VOICES**
>
> Each day this week, pick a situation in which you will listen to another person's voice and evaluate it clinically.
>
> - What features do you hear that you can describe?
> - If you have an understanding of the GRBAS scale, can you rate the speaker in your mind? Use the table below to record your rating; this is also in the accompanying web page.
> - How does this person's voice differ from the person they're speaking to?

	G (overall grade)	B (breathiness)	R (roughness)	A (asthenia or weakness)	S (strain)
Speaker 1					
Speaker 2					
Speaker 3					
Speaker 4					
Speaker 5					

REFERENCES

Gottliebson, R. O., Lee, L., Weinrich, B. & Sanders, J. (2007) Voice Problems of Future Speech-Language Pathologists *Journal of Voice* 21 (6) 699–704 https://doi.org/10.1016/j.jvoice.2006.07.003

Joseph, B. E., Joseph, A. M. & Jacob, T. M. (2020) Vocal Fatigue – Do Young Speech-Language Pathologists Practice What They Preach? *Journal of Voice* 34 (4) 647.e1–647.e5 https://doi.org/10.1016/j.jvoice.2018.11.015

Knickerbocker, K., Bryan, C. & Ziegler, A. (2021) Phonogenic Voice Problems among Speech-Language Pathologists in Synchronous Telepractice: An Overview and Recommendations. *Seminars in Speech and Language* 42 (1) 73–84 https://doi.org/10.1055/s-0040-1722754

Rumbach, A. F., Dallaston, K. & Hill, A. E. (2021) Student Perceptions of Factors that Influence Clinical Competency in Voice. *International Journal of Speech-Language Pathology* 23 (2) https://doi.org/10.1080/17549507.2020.1737733

Searl, J. & Dargin, T. (2021) Voice and Lifestyle Behaviors of Speech-Language Pathology Students: Impact of History Gathering Method of Self-Reported Data. *Journal of Voice* 35 (1) 158.e9–158.e20 https://doi.org/10.1016/j.jvoice.2019.08.014

Van Lierde, K. M., D'haeseleer, E., Wuyts, F. L., De Ley, S., Geldof, R., De Vuyst, J. & Sofie, C. (2010) The Objective Vocal Quality, Vocal Risk Factors, Vocal Complaints, and Corporal Pan in Dutch Female Students Training to be Speech-Language Pathologists During the 4 Years of Study. *Journal of Voice* 24 (5) 592–598 https://doi.org/10.1016/j.jvoice.2008.12.011

Warhurst, S., Madill, C., McCabe, P., Heard, R. & Yiu, E. (2012) The Vocal Clarity of Female Speech-Language Pathology Students: An Exploratory Study. *Journal of Voice* 26 (1) 63–68 https://doi.org/10.1016/j.jvoice.2010.10.008

Chapter 3

"DOING" VOICE THERAPY

Wrapped around specific therapy exercises are several general principles of "how to do" voice therapy which are presented across 10 tips in this chapter. We will consider how to facilitate change in our clients through collaborative working, tenderness, and a spirit of inclusivity and openness to diversity. Thinking about the different possible outcomes of voice therapy guides us towards how we prove our therapy is effective and helps us manage times where progress is moving more slowly. All these skills influence the many roles we inhabit and the roles of teacher, coach, and problem solver are considered specifically. Many of the tips are not exclusive to a voice caseload but are applied to voice as the client group we currently share.

TIP 4 – UNDERSTANDING CHANGE

We're only three tips in and already you have vocal experimentation under your belt. What facilitated or hindered this? Was vocal rest easier during a journey alone to work or placement, for example, but harder when others were around? What did you prioritise? Your vocal care, your sense of commitment to the experiment, or internal and external pressures to engage with others? If you prioritised vocal care because you understood its importance, you've mirrored a potential client. If you completed the experiment through curiosity about what might happen, you've mirrored a potential client. Can you guess the response if you found it hard to resist internal or external pressures? Yes – you've mirrored a potential client! The takeaway message here is that different clients react to SLT guidance in different ways and in some you may see a reflection of yourself.

The challenges of voice change

van Leer et al. (2008) ask a very pertinent question: "Why do some voice patients diligently practise their daily voice exercises, whereas others return only to provide reasons for not doing so? Why do some overcome struggles in changing vocal health behaviours, whereas others give up at the first sign of difficulty?" (p. 689). There are several internal and external reasons for this. For some clients, the short-term investment in therapy practice promotes engagement (White & Carding, 2020) where others may admit that voice therapy is hard (van Leer & Connor, 2010) and indeed it can be. Human behaviour means we often don't make change in a straightforward, A-to-B, fashion and you may relate to this if you've ever set a resolution to become fitter, healthier, or more organised and then found yourself not progressing as you'd hoped.

van Leer and Connor (2010) identified the following challenges for clients attending voice therapy:

- remembering to practise each day
- remembering to use the target voice beyond specific practice activities

- being able to make independent judgements about their voice when not with the clinician (also known as "being your own therapist")
- needing increased cognitive effort to think about the voice
- practising without feeling embarrassed, particularly if others can hear
- feeling like the target voice is not unnatural

The self-development activities in Tip 2 should help you empathise with the challenge of remembering to practise and when you practise the voice-specific exercises in Tips 14, 22, 23, 29, and 32 you may also empathise with the challenges of self-evaluation and needing to overcome your inhibitions.

Internal influences on change

Models of behavioural change recognise that clients attend with different levels of readiness to make change, and this readiness (or not) will influence our therapy recommendations. Our clients might strongly desire a less hoarse voice, but they may not be ready to stop smoking or practise exercises three times a day! Understanding whether clients are not yet ready to think about doing things differently (pre-contemplation), beginning to think about it (contemplation), starting to dip a toe in the water of change (preparation), creating an early routine (action), or sustaining lasting changes (maintenance) ensures we mould our therapy plans to our client needs (van Leer et al., 2008).

As well as guiding therapy plans, understanding behavioural change allows us to be more forgiving towards clients who are experiencing slower progress, which is further explored in Tip 12. Rather than judging clients as non-committed to therapy, or blaming ourselves for not being able to persuade clients to follow our advice, might they be at a different stage of readiness to change to where we think they are? Understanding the non-linear nature of change can also be reassuring for clients caught between their expectations of therapy and the actual reality, so be prepared to explain the theory of change to them.

Additionally, Burleson's (2009) model of supportive communication highlights the influence of our client's ability or readiness to take on advice. You might be able to think of a time where you weren't ready to hear advice even if you knew it to be wise and relevant. This is true for our clients too – our guidance might be of high quality but if they are not ready to take this on board or are unable to fully process it, making change becomes more difficult.

External influences on change

Moving beyond general readiness to change, the Health Belief Model accounts for external influences on change including demographic and psychological influences, such as class, age, and peer or group pressure. The model also recognises that we weigh up the perceptions around susceptibility and severity of a potential disease (in this case dysphonia) alongside the perceived benefits and barriers to taking action (Abraham & Sheehan, 2005). For our clients, this may mean an increased likelihood of following vocal health recommendations and engagement with practice by a performer who believes their career to be at risk and can see the value in SLT, compared with a low chance of vocal health advice being followed by a client who believes smoking does not cause cancer and whose social network includes several fellow smokers.

Situating voice therapy within a social cognitive therapy (SCT) framework brings a further influential layer of "in the moment" decisions (van Leer, 2021). Adapting the smoking example above, we might work with someone who, through your education, better understands the health risks associated with smoking and has the internal drive to stop but still accepts the offer of a cigarette when socialising at the end of a stressful week. This doesn't mean they're not ready to take any action towards stopping smoking, but that achieving their goal might be made more difficult in certain circumstances. Accompanying Abraham and Sheehan's chapter on the Health Belief Model, Connor and Norman (2005) provide a good overview of several health behaviour theories for onward learning.

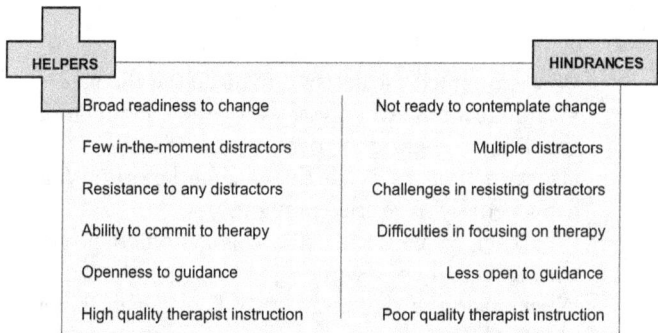

Figure 1 Summary of helpers and hindrances to behavioural change

Figure 1 shows a summary of client helpers and hindrances to change and I'd encourage you to keep this in mind in your practice. Can you identify clients for whom the helpers have combined to create a smooth-sailing therapy experience and clients for whom therapy is challenging them to concentrate on aspects of voice they find difficult or unfamiliar?

Client change is facilitated by working collaboratively so head to the next tip once you've reflected on your own change through self-development activity 8. Tips 9 and 10 consider the influence of our communication on therapeutic interactions and change more deeply.

> **SELF-DEVELOPMENT ACTIVITY 8 – REFLECTING ON YOUR OWN CHANGE**
>
> Can you think of a change you've tried to make? It could be starting a new gym programme, creating a more effective study schedule, or varying what you have for lunch.... Whether you consider the change to be successful or not, use the questions below to reflect on your experience.

- What was the change you were making?
- What prompted the decision to make the change?
- Was there a time when you were pre-contemplation and didn't recognise the need to change at all?
- Had you tried to make this change before? What happened if you've tried previously?
- What helped you with this change, whether you tried it recently or a while ago?
- What made the change more difficult, even if you ultimately managed to make the change?
- Can you see what stage, or stages, you've progressed through in relation to this change?
- Were there times when you were keen for the final outcome(s) but found the change difficult to maintain?
- Did any "in the moment" factors influence your change?
- How can you use these reflections to benefit your practice?

TIP 5 – WORKING COLLABORATIVELY

Historically, the terms "adherence" and "compliance" were used to judge how much clients followed our advice and although they imply a hierarchical relationship in which clients should simply obey the SLT, you'll still see the words in contemporary research (e.g. Ebersole et al., 2017; Marques Torbes et al., 2020; Slavych et al., 2021; van Leer, 2021). No study offers a definition of adherence but good adherence is often positively linked with consistent attendance and successful outcomes (Marques Torbes et al., 2020; Rubino & Abbott, in press), and conversely non-adherence is attributed to clients who stop attending or do not improve. Rather than viewing non-adherence as client rebellion, can we reframe this more constructively? Can we incorporate our knowledge of change (Tip 4), be more understanding of therapeutic challenges, and then use collaborative problem solving to identify how change can be facilitated?

Although there can certainly be gains if clients practise as we advise, we are not in a position of authority from where we can blame the client if they do not follow our rules. Healthcare has moved on from positioning clients as needing to be saved and professionals as those who will do the saving – instead viewing therapy as something we do *with* clients rather than *to* them equalises client and clinician contributions to therapy so neither party has greater power over the other. An equal therapist–client dyad brings an openness to the relationship, gives us permission to not have all the answers, and contributes to clients feeling heard.

Additionally, asking voice clients to modify their routines or lifestyle, adjust to lifelong difficulties, look inwards to their stresses, or consider adaptations to their jobs are all significant changes so approaching them from a position of unity is more helpful than from a position of "therapist knows best". Evidence-based practice (EBP) draws on the most current research evidence but also builds on therapist experience and client opinion, and Mannix's (2021) tender conversational skills (Tip 7) will support you here. Can you be truly open to hearing what the client has to say as part of working collaboratively? Truly acknowledging the client views will be important when you come to decide what therapy to offer, or not, and this is addressed in Tip 18.

Behlau et al.'s (in press) coaching questions can help elicit useful client data and include: "what is driving you to get a good voice?", "what would be an acceptable timeframe for you to show improvements in your voice?", "what has been the most useful thing until now for you to improve your voice?", and "what have you learned so far about yourself and the way you use your voice?" Asking such questions reinforces your interest in your client's experience, encouraging clients to buy in to therapy and take on responsibility for their therapy.

Further supporting the mindset of coaching questions and collaborative working is solution-focused brief therapy (SFBT) (Burns, 2005). The nature of assessment and the purpose of therapy often shine a light on the client's problem but SFBT, as the name suggests, focuses on the solution. It invites our clients to describe times when their problem isn't present, identify what is working well for them in those moments, and subsequently use those existing strengths and strategies to move forwards towards a solution. Such questions automatically invite your clients in to a therapy partnership and I would encourage you to incorporate solution-focused language in your conversations alongside exploration of the issues at hand.

TIP 6 – THE CLIENT AS ACTIVE AGENT

The two previous tips, understanding change and working collaboratively, ask us to move away from a directive, authoritarian approach to therapy but if progress is almost exclusively reliant on practise outside of therapy appointments (van Leer, 2021), how do we nurture client responsibility for change? This is influenced by a combination of self-regulation, agency, and self-efficacy as seen in Figure 2.

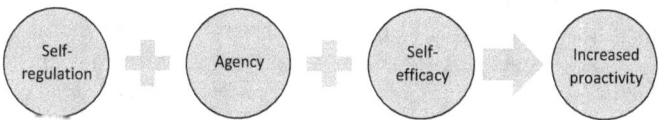

Figure 2   The social-cognitive concepts contributing to client responsibility for practice

Self-regulation

Self-regulation is the ability to manage our own behaviours and, with respect to change, requires clients to be motivated, monitor different situations and feelings, and have willpower. Although motivation for practice may be aided by employment (Slavych et al., 2021) or higher voice demand and higher self-rating scores (Ebersole et al., 2017), all clients should assume some responsibility for their independent practise which might include inhibiting voice use, practising your recommended exercises, or maintaining the skills they have developed through therapy. Behlau et al.'s (in press) coaching questions can help again to maximise a client's potential, particularly in asking: "what would be the best way to motivate you to do the exercises?" or "what alternative options do you have when you do not have time to do the exercises?".

Agency

Agency is the ability to take on responsibility for our own change and some clients may need to create, with your support, a new perspective that their voice should be cared for. Once clients acknowledge their part in short-term voice care and long-term voice change, working with the voice comes more easily. It doesn't fully eradicate the possibility of challenges but envisioning the possibility of change generates a closer connection with the overall process.

Self-efficacy

Self-efficacy is our internal belief about our ability to complete a task which, in turn, influences whether we attempt a task and how much effort we put into it. When we introduce clients to new tasks, many of them are SLT-specific, which may bring feelings of being daunted, anxious, or hesitant. Indeed, van Leer and Connor (2015) confirmed that some voice exercises are just plain weird and beliefs about voice practice at the start of voice therapy can significantly predict whether clients actually practise (van Leer, 2021). Self-efficacy is not a fixed construct, however, and can be enhanced through successful mastery of a task, watching others complete the tasks, feeling physically comfortable when practising, and hearing encouragement from others (van Leer et al., 2008). Videos of therapist modelling, client-as-model, and peer testimonials (van Leer & Connor, 2015) also increase self-efficacy, as do digital reminders accompanied by realistic goals and positive self-talk (van Leer, 2021). As you practise, which of the self-efficacy supports could you use so mastery of one skill feeds in to belief about potential mastery of others?

A note about your self-efficacy

Although this tip focuses on developing client self-regulation, agency, and self-efficacy, this is an ideal moment to reflect on self-regulation, agency, and self-efficacy in relation to your own voice skills. Remembering that Rumbach et al.'s (2021) SLT students developed their confidence through practice, make sure you create time and space to practise voice exercises before demonstrating these in the clinic. Belief in your clinical skills will change your posture, your demeanour, and increase your internal confidence in managing any unexpected challenges. If *you're* confident in demonstrating the task, your client is more likely to follow you, and if you appear less confident or demonstrate cautiously, the client may not fully understand what is expected of them. Even experienced therapists may feel some mild uncertainty about a new therapy approach but self-belief allows them to take the steps in trying out new skills, and I encourage you to do the same.

> **SELF-DEVELOPMENT ACTIVITY 9 – EXTENDING YOUR CLINIC LINGO**
>
> As you work with different clinicians, you will hear phrases which capture an instruction or feedback particularly well and replicating these phrases yourself can increase your confidence in therapeutic interactions and beliefs around self-efficacy. Note any useful phrases you hear as an expanding resource for your practice.

TIP 7 – CULTIVATING TENDER CONVERSATIONS

This chapter was initially titled "having difficult conversations", influenced by the terminology students, colleagues, and I have previously used to describe therapeutic discussions which involve careful navigation and perhaps discomfort for both client and therapist. During my writing I have been introduced to Mannix's (2021) more appropriate terminology of tender conversations, which rightly highlights that "labelling conversations as difficult carry a sense of negativity and self-defence… [conflicting with] the "I'm here for you mindset" (p. 37). Academic counselling texts will furnish you with the theory of person-centredness in healthcare but Mannix (2021) is a very readable introduction to the importance of listening skills. We don't always need to find a solution to a problem – just being with clients can exude a spirit of support and on some occasions will be experienced as more supportive than had we offered specific advice.

Tender conversational skills aren't reserved for sensitive or potentially painful topics though – as you observe others at work and as you develop your own experience you will notice that tender skills are everywhere. They permeate your initial contact with clients, they are seamlessly interwoven with your therapy and remain knitted in practice as you discuss discharge.

Developing skills in facilitating tender conversations enables us to ask about a client's mental well-being, explore the difficult work dynamics contributing to the dysphonia, gather more information about erratic menstrual cycles, and explain the importance of smoking or alcohol cessation without a sense of judgement, and all of this is done without clients noticing whether you are in "counselling mode" or "instructional mode". Sometimes, when a client and I have discussed wider challenges in life, they will comment "this is just like having my own therapist". They use the term therapist to refer to a counsellor or other professional supporting mental well-being but I smile because for me, the clue is in my professional title and I *am* a therapist! I'm not a fully trained counsellor but I do have counselling skills and I am always ready to listen.

Western society is increasingly acknowledging the importance of positive mental health and the value of talking about our worries, but clients will still only share what feels personally comfortable. Sharing little does not necessarily reflect their level of trust with you but instead how comfortable they are pursuing previously unspoken topics. It is one thing to think about how difficult work is or inwardly acknowledge an abusive relationship, for example, but quite another to speak about it. Putting our troubles "out there" can heighten their reality and such acknowledgement can feel frightening or unsettling. I can acknowledge that to cope with particularly difficult circumstances I've sought professional counselling but have occasionally omitted details when it felt too vulnerable to speak about the full experience and I should know that counselling is a safe space! Being privileged to such information can place us in a position where we know more about a client's life than some of their family, friends, or colleagues, and such conversations deserve respect and active listening.

> **SELF-DEVELOPMENT ACTIVITY 10 – REFLECTING ON YOUR OWN TENDER CONVERSATIONS**
>
> - Can you think of a time when you limited your description of an experience?
> - Do you know why you only shared part of your experience?
> - Did you share the rest of the details at a later date?
> - How can you take this experience in to your practice?

Introducing tender conversations

So how do we introduce tender subjects in our clinical conversations? Clients are likely to be taken aback if we simply ask: "how is your mental health?" but providing a context makes the rationale for my enquiry explicit and I might say something similar to:

> *"So far we've spoken about influences on your voice such as smoking or how much you use your voice at work, and some of the other things which can have a bearing on your voice are stress, worries or anxieties. I wonder if there's anything either very present for you, or niggles at the back of your mind which are causing upset?"*

This gives space for clients to share significant life pressures as well as seemingly unimportant worries. If you are unfamiliar or uncomfortable with introducing tender conversations, I would recommend writing a script like the one above, and then practising it with friends or family members.

Onward navigation through tender conversations

Although I am now experienced in listening to clients' distress, some conversations still have an emotional impact on me and you may also experience an inner unsettlement because you, too, are human. Silence provides space for clients to talk and encourages us to truly listen, and so I invite you to reflect on your comfort with silence. Are you able to sit with someone else and feel no pressure to say anything or do you feel obliged to make comment? Perhaps you're very chatty and like to talk, perhaps sometimes you forget to listen, or perhaps you're worried you don't know what to say so fill the gap before thinking about your response.

If you tried the voice conservation task in self-development activity 5, your reflections on silence can help you here. Our tolerance of silence may be influenced by the caseload, our knowledge and experience but, as SLTs or SLTs-in-training, this is an important skill. If silences feel difficult for you, try practising some. You could resist the urge to give advice to a friend, replacing this with a reflective *"that sounds difficult"* to invite further comment, or you could nod to show support without offering immediate advice. Even if your toes are curling a little as you develop comfort with tender conversations (and that's ok because your clients can't see your toes!), remember the privileged position you're in when offering a fully active listening ear to your clients. Providing space for others can be really powerful and clients may cry during your conversations as a release of emotion and perhaps as a reflection of the safety they feel in your presence.

> **SELF-DEVELOPMENT ACTIVITY 11 – REFLECTING ON YOUR EXPERIENCES OF BEING HEARD**
>
> - Can you think of a conversation where you felt truly heard? What did the other person or people do to leave you with that feeling?
> - Can you think of a conversation where you did not feel heard? What did your listener(s) do in this situation to give that feeling?
> - What can you take from these conversations into your practice with respect to what you intend to do/do not intend to do?

Confidentiality

Discussion of tender conversations would be incomplete without a note on confidentiality. As you will undoubtedly hear sensitive and personal information during practice, it should go without saying that none of this information is shared with anyone other than another healthcare professional for whom the data are relevant. You should additionally seek your client's consent to divulge information to their general practitioner (GP) or a mental health practitioner, unless there are significant concerns regarding their immediate safety which takes precedence over consent.

TIP 8 – REMOTE VS. FACE-TO-FACE THERAPY

At the time of writing, there is a boom in providing therapy online in response to a global pandemic, though readers in five or ten years' time may be well-accustomed to a combination of in-person and remote therapy. Prior to COVID-19, remote therapy was largely used to provide healthcare to communities who were unable to travel to clinics or for whom travelling was excessive, but social restrictions aiming to prevent virus spread allowed us to see the full value of telehealth and accelerate the speed with which it was adopted. Not only does telehealth keep clinicians and clients safe in the current health climate, there is greater client convenience with reduced travel costs (Doll et al., 2021). A link to professional guidelines, produced by the Royal College of Speech and Language Therapists (RCSLT), is at the end of this chapter.

Looking after the remote client voice

Early voice research in the context of COVID-19 suggests the recent surge in homeworking has led to vocal tract discomfort and dysphonia (Kenny, in press) and I'd be surprised if these Irish results weren't mirrored elsewhere in the general population. Although we can't be certain that homeworking is responsible for the difficulties, the fact that 85% of those with new-onset dysphonia developed this since the start of restrictions strongly suggests a link. Temporary home offices are unlikely to have vocal heath at the heart of the design – poor seating posture, for example, can compromise breath support and lead to muscular tension, both widespread in the body and more specifically in the head and neck. Given the recent benefits of homeworking, this looks set to become more established practice and so we need to ensure our clients' environment and work demands permit good vocal care rather than increasing the risk of discomfort and dysphonia (Kenny, in press; Kishbaugh et al., in press).

The challenges of conducting online voice assessment and therapy

Challenges exist for both our clients and us. Some homeworkers may have office furniture which supports their posture and head positioning in front of the camera, while others may be using a mobile phone balanced against a vase. An upright posture in a tension-free body may not be possible if a client is looking towards a device that is lower than them (on a coffee table, for instance) and the altered neck positioning may impact on their vocal performance. Unable to control the client's lighting, background noise, the communication device being used, and the position of this, we may have a distorted perspective of our client's attempts at specific activities. A bird's eye view or a worm's eye view is not the equivalent of what we would normally see in clinic!

Sustained sounds are not always fully registered by a computer microphone and poor positioning of the device may alter the client's posture, reducing the opportunity for you to modify their positioning like we could do in-clinic. Furthermore, some clients may have excellent broadband connection so there is no buffering or freezing, whilst others may experience frequent disruptions meaning the camera needs to be off to retain a connection. A final aspect of voice care that can't be provided online is any manual therapy such as circumlaryngeal manipulation.

Looking after the therapist voice

When we work in-person, our proximity to clients informs us how loud our voice needs to be but without this cue during online therapy, we may find ourselves projecting as if our voices are travelling right to our clients' houses when in fact we only need our voices to reach the microphone a few inches away. Non-verbal cues are less visible and we may attempt to compensate by expressing our "likeability" through other means, including altered and possibly maladaptive use of the voice. Minimising the risk of voice difficulties is possible through limiting the number of telehealth sessions, resting the voice at other times, drinking plenty of water, configuring speaker and microphone settings to minimise sound distortion, using vocal warm-ups and cool-downs, and accessing support for any growing fatigue, strain, or hoarseness (Knickerbocker et al., 2021). This guidance from Knickerbocker and colleagues is very applicable to clients working from home and using remote communication platforms, and the British Voice Association also has information for maintaining a healthy virtual voice, with advice suitable for both clients and therapists. The link is at the end of this chapter.

TIP 9 – A BLEND OF SLT PERSONALITIES

Although we know that a good therapist–client match is important (van Leer and Connor, 2010) and a low-quality therapeutic alliance risks clients ending therapy prematurely (Sylvestre & Gobeil, 2020), we don't yet know how client, therapist, and service delivery factors specifically combine to influence progress (Eastwood et al., 2015). In this tip, let's take a look at your role in shaping positive outcomes.

The different faces of SLT

Under the title of speech and language therapist, we'll adopt the roles of teacher, counsellor, model of good voice care, coach, and problem solver as in Figure 3.

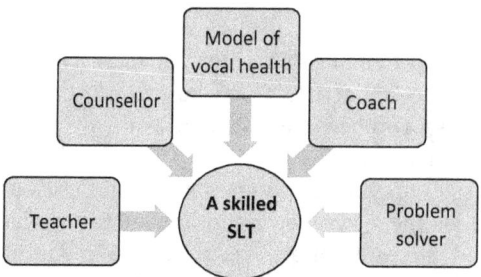

Figure 3 The different roles of a speech and language therapist

Self-development activity 4 encouraged you to develop your own vocal care and become a model of vocal health, Tip 5 included coaching questions as a means of encouraging change, and Tip 7 highlighted the important qualities in your counselling role so this tip will consider the other two roles of teacher and problem-solver. The overarching role of a reflective practitioner will support your development in all other roles.

The therapist as teacher

Madill et al. (2020) identify two stages of voice therapy: *pre-practice* and *practice*. The former is clinic-based with verbal information and modelling to guide your clients towards the target voice quality. When providing explanations, the quality of our information needs to be high and tailored to the individual so they are able to digest this. We might use short and simple instructions, rather than long and complex utterances, we can provide information before or during a client's attempt, we can refer to movements or metaphors ("it's as if you're yawning") or we can provide information about specific vocal mechanisms, such as vocal fold vibration (Madill et al., 2020). Your specific explanations about how to complete the task will be supplemented by the rationale for the activity.

When clients understand why they are doing what they are doing they are more likely to engage with our advice (White & Carding, 2020) and I have certainly found this to be true in my practice. I often share snippets of research, explained in layperson's terms, so clients are aware I am drawing on an evidence base for my decisions – each time you read a journal article, think how you could summarise the results so you become skilled at distilling research for a non-academic audience.

Alongside providing our rationale for decisions, clients may also ask their own questions, influenced by what they've sourced on the internet and via social media. Unfortunately, not all online information is consistently accurate or accessible for the lay reader (Dueppen et al., 2019; Alwani et al. 2021; Doruk et al., 2020) so be ready to evaluate the information clients bring to you. Be particularly careful about tabloid reports which have not applied critical analysis to breaking research and instead sensationalise new treatments beyond their actual worth.

In the practice phase, which is unsupervised and situated away from the clinic, clients use pre-practice knowledge and repetitions of exercises to build their skills as an important part of generalisation (van Leer, 2021; Rubino & Abbott, in press). Although therapy is separated by Madill et al. into two distinct phases, in reality pre-practice and practice phases overlap so while clients are practising one set of exercises at home or work, we may be teaching them something else in clinic.

The therapist as problem solver

Although our therapy plans are created in good faith that they target the problem at hand, it is rare for a plan never to be tweaked in response to client feedback or the realities of practice. Here we can look to Iwarsson (2015) to expand our problem solving skills.

Adapting the environment (cue-altering)

Advice in isolation may be insufficient to change vocal habits so a wider perspective, which considers the context in which the client is attempting to implement your advice, is required. Instead of a broad suggestion of reduced occupational voice use, for example, you may need an activity which identifies where in a client's work schedule they have opportunities for voice conservation. Alternatively, you and your client may need to construct a more vocally supportive home environment which could include discussion around safe calling of the family for dinner, alternative ways of building in character to bedtime stories, or how to continue university socialising without harming the voice.

The client as problem solver (cognitive activation)

In early therapy sessions, problem solving will often be therapist-led with an aim of clients becoming increasingly independent during therapy and then assuming the responsibility for problem solving at the point of discharge. Although we don't want clients to struggle long term with voice practice, the cognitive effort needed to navigate the occasional challenge increases motor learning and ultimately self-efficacy (Tip 6). I love the moments where clients pause before attempting phonation or a particular movement as it means they've decided the optimal conditions haven't been laid for the voice activity. This in-the-moment, proactive problem solving is evidence they're embedding their voice skills, becoming their own therapist, and moving towards independent self-management (van Leer & Connor, 2010).

Negative practice

The long-term goal of therapy is usually to move away from the difficulty but we can exploit unwanted phonation or voice technique as a contrast to the target and as an additional learning opportunity. Being able to switch between desired and unwanted phonation under the client's own volition develops vocal control and reiterates the different physical conditions leading to each. Iwarsson (2015) cautions that negative practice must be done in a playful but sensitive manner as producing an unwanted sound may not be a comfortable experience for some clients.

The therapist as artist and scientist

Voicework blends both art and science. Our understanding of the technicalities of the voice and our critical thinking around the evidence base support the scientist in us, and our use of imagination, imagery, and encouragement for clients to feel the voice as well as hear it supports our inner artist. For example, if I explain the use of top up breaths with reference to inhalations, exhalations, and the respiratory system, and ask a client to identify where top-up breaths could be using utterances of increasing length (Tip 24), I'm drawing on a scientific approach. Alternatively, if I describe the cyclical process of breathing as "riding the wave of the breath" with the crest of the wave representing replenished breath support, this artistic approach guides clients away from viewing inhalation and exhalation as a discrete two-part process which can contribute to overthinking the breath.

We may have personal tendencies towards one perspective – I think I'm more artist than scientist – and our clients may also have their own preferences (van Leer, 2021) so to decide which approach may be beneficial, follow the kind of terminology your clients use. Be open to using both a scientific and artistic approach though – I'm still learning new skills, some of which fit with my more natural artistic approach and some of which develop me as a scientific practitioner.

TIP 10 – GIVING FEEDBACK

In order to learn, we all need feedback. As a student you receive feedback on university assignments and your clinical skills on placement. If you are already qualified, a mentor may offer feedback as you discuss your plans and they observe your sessions. The same is true for clients – they need feedback to learn and be guided to increasingly accurate production of the intended sound or voice quality.

Your feedback will be influenced by both what you hear and what you see. In your early development as a voice therapist, it will be easier to notice the significant changes but with increasing experience you will tune into more subtle shifts in the voice and markers of change. Sometimes a mere flicker of a facial expression catches my attention and is evidence of independent client thinking.

Enhancing feedback quality

High-quality feedback is timely, accurate, specific, and collaborative. Let's look at each of these qualities in more detail.

Timely

Without needing to comment on every attempt or piece of conversation, you should provide timely feedback during or after an attempt. Leaving a client to practise without direction reduces the opportunity to change successive attempts and as moments pass it becomes increasingly difficult for us and clients to recall the vocal nuances in previous conversations or activities.

Accurate

There is little point in providing inaccurate feedback. At best, it doesn't further your client's learning and, at worst, it provides confusing information which hinders progress. If a client thinks their attempt is appropriate but it isn't, they will continue to practise inaccurately. Although it feels good to be able to congratulate a client on a clearer or more efficient voice, do also address the less successful attempts. You could say: *"I can see your determination to achieve this sound but that's contributing to your whole body becoming involved with a bigger breath and raised shoulders. Can you try that again and see if you can allow your shoulders to settle down? Watch me again..."*

Specific

As well as judging whether task attempts were nearer to, or further away from, the target, client's also need to know why you have made that judgement. A binary evaluation of whether a client's attempt was correct or incorrect is only partially informative as it doesn't capture the scale of accuracy or inaccuracy. For instance, a sound may not reach the ultimate desired quality but it might be 80% on its way there. Is that a correct or incorrect attempt then? Rather than opting for an "either or" split, or saying "good" as an acknowledgement of an attempt, more specific, helpful, feedback could be:

> *"I noticed how you paused before trying the sound and that's great – you seemed to have an intuitive sense that diving straight in wouldn't work."*

or

> *"Those extra breaths really helped you to not be out of breath by the end of the sentence and so your voice was less strained."*

Collaborative

Tip 5 highlighted the importance of collaborative working and for complete voice evaluation your observations should be complemented by what your client hears, feels, and locates (Tip 23). A clear voice quality with a client report of mild effort has scope for development but an audibly clear voice quality, supported by a client-reported feeling of vocal ease, is a great success. "What did you think?" is a useful starting question but asking "what did you hear?" or "what sensations did you notice?" or "how did that compare to the previous sound?" invites more refined observations. The development of awareness in Tip 22 will aid your client to tune in to subtle signals, deepen their learning and develop more accurate self-evaluation which are all aspects of unsupervised home practice (Tip 9). If you think you might forget to ask your client for their opinion as you concentrate on conducting your session, do include questions to elicit client feedback in your session plans as a memory aid.

Alternative feedback

Verbal comments are likely to be the most commonly used form of feedback in your sessions as they are readily accessible but you should also consider comparisons of pre-therapy audio recordings with in-therapy attempts and recordings made at the point of discharge, video-recordings to consider the wider body aspects of voicework, and visually displayed feedback from acoustic analysis.

TIP 11 – DEFINING OUTCOMES

Even at the start of therapy, we'll be thinking ahead to the final outcome. What do we want to achieve, what do we want our clients to do that they're not able to do now, and how can we measure this to prove our therapy has been successful? Any outcome evaluation needs a "before" and "after" value for comparison – there is little merit in a client completing a self-rating assessment at the end of therapy and being pleased with low scores if we don't know the original ratings. Pre-therapy and post-therapy comparisons can also be captured through repeated laryngeal evaluation, repeated acoustic and perceptual assessment, and therapist use of a recognised outcome tool such as Therapy Outcome Measures (TOMs) (Enderby et al., 2006). Using the dysphonia-specific section of TOMs, therapists rate the client's abilities on four different categories: impairment, activity, participation, and well-being/distress. Therapy may facilitate changes across all four sections but may improve on well-being and activity, for example, even if the impairment changes little. The rationale for these data is three-fold: to demonstrate the provision of effective therapy as individual clinicians, to prove that as service we have a positive impact on our immediate community, and to confirm that as a profession we're deserving of public funding for clinical practice and research.

Client-generated outcomes

Varying client perceptions of a positive outcome mean it can be difficult to objectively assess success (Gillespie & Gartner-Schmidt, 2018). A client with vocal fatigue from long working hours might realistically hope for an end to their fatigue, a client with recurring laryngeal papillomas (Tip 37) might also want a cure but recurrence means full and immediate resolution is not possible, and for a client with inducible laryngeal obstruction (Tip 33) being able to manage symptoms as they arise might be their desired success. Your first data-gathering session can be concluded with the very revealing question of: "how will you know it has been worthwhile coming to SLT?". Not only does that encourage the client to look ahead and imagine their outcome at the point of discharge, it also provides you with information around client expectations.

Voice-related outcomes

As well as considering what outcome the client desires, we also need to consider what outcomes are possible in the context of the medical diagnosis, the evidence around the diagnosis, and client engagement with therapy. Combining these data generates the following possible outcomes:

- your client not only regains pre-morbid voice quality but therapy enhances their voice, building a stronger voice for the future
- your client regains pre-morbid voice quality and is able to return to all previous communication situations
- your client achieves a voice which does not reach their pre-morbid voice quality but is adequate for their needs and is the optimal possible quality given the client's diagnosis
- there is little or no discernible change in the voice and there may be limitations on communication opportunities

You can have these possible outcomes in mind at the start of therapy and review the direction of progress as therapy ensues. Bear in mind that clients may change their desired level of function as they become aware of what therapy entails. For some clients this may mean reducing their expectations while others will increase their hopes – I worked with a singer who started therapy to address her vocal fold nodules with the hope of achieving a good voice but progressed to aiming for an awesome voice once she realised the potential of therapy.

Function-related outcomes

The outcomes above focus on the presence or absence of voice changes but these do not specify the level of function which is situated in the context of our client's vocal demands. For instance, a return to normal voice quality which existed pre-nodules might be success for a client with low vocal load but returning to a pre-nodular voice quality may be insufficient for a teacher to permit full functioning in an occupational environment. Conversely, a client with presbyphonia is unlikely to return to their voice quality of 20 years ago due to vocal fold atrophy but supporting them to achieve maximum functioning within their individual context is more realistic.

Discharge

In Tips 6 and 9 we started to think about the client becoming their own therapist. The ability to transfer skills from a clinic setting to everyday conversational speech can be an important influence on discharge (Gillespie & Gartner-Schmidt, 2018) though agreement to conclude therapy doesn't need to wait until clients are using their new voice skills 100% of the time. Being able to manage their voice independently still permits discharge, even if voicework is a lifetime investment for those reliant on their voice for work or leisure.

Gillespie and Gartner-Schmidt (2018) are clear that discharge criteria are distinguished from the number and duration of therapy sessions – this means some clients may be discharged after three appointments of 40 minutes where other clients may require eight or more sessions lasting 50 minutes to "future-proof" their voice against further difficulties. In reality, a limit on public health spending, a ceiling on the number of available sessions funded by an insurance company, or the client's own ability to self-fund may influence the number of possible sessions but discharge criteria for gold standard care should not include pre-determined quantification of therapy input.

Discharge should also always be collaborative and incorporate client evaluation as well as our assessment of voice. For many clients discharge is a positive experience as it is evidence of progress but for others it may carry a sense of disappointment or frustration if therapy hasn't given them what they'd hoped for, or external circumstances prevented ongoing attendance.

Wider outcomes

In addition to the client-related outcomes, successful therapy has the power to impact more widely as in Figure 4.

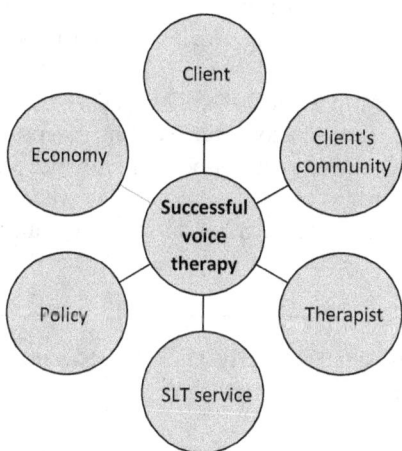

Figure 4 The potential wider community positively impacted by SLT input

Starting at the top of Figure 4 and moving clockwise, a client with a positive experience of voice therapy will feel the impact at an individual level and if they spread the word of the benefit of SLT, there is positive impact within their immediate community – not only do they believe that SLT is valuable, so too do their friends, family, and work colleagues. This enhanced view of SLT may help those later referred to voice therapy and some of my clients have shared vocal advice with family, friends, and colleagues which prompted others to seek help.

Successful therapy outcomes also impact positively on us and that doesn't go away. I experience as much pleasure now observing the impact of my therapy as I did as a newly qualified therapist, and individual positive outcomes have a ripple effect as they confirm that local financial investment in services, and indeed our wider profession, brings results.

More rarely our input with individual clients leads to policy change, though recognition of our value with particular voice user groups can slowly contribute to policy shifts – growing recognition of the risk of voice difficulties for teachers by an education authority, for example, may lead to local change regarding working conditions or the vocal support offered.

Finally, our input can be economically beneficial. Therapy which allows clients to continue working means continued tax revenue and reduced costs associated with sick leave cover in professions, such as teaching and nursing, where an employee on sick leave and the member of staff covering the role are both paid.

> **SELF-DEVELOPMENT ACTIVITY 12 – CONSIDERING THE OUTCOMES OF YOUR THERAPY**
>
> As you work with different clients, identify what difference(s) you are making. Is this for your client, their listeners or wider community, you, your service, policy, or the economy? You may be providing a benefit in more than one of these categories! Use the table in the online Self-development Activities resource to record your thoughts as evidence of the wide-reaching impact your therapy is having.

Client initials	Occupation	Speaker (client) impact	Listener impact	Economic impact

TIP 12 – WHEN PROGRESS SLOWS

Tips 4, 5, 6, 9, and 10 specifically focused on nurturing client progress, and it would be logical to think that by following all the suggestions, success will follow but what if it doesn't? How do we establish the reasons behind slower progress, and how can we respond, bearing in mind that in addition to the severity and duration of the problem, the rate of voice change can be altered by both therapist and client factors? The prompt questions below encourage reflection on the different reasons for slow progress.

Therapist factors

Is my therapy targeting the most pressing concern?

Our initial plan should be clearly linked to the most pressing concern which emerged from our case history and assessment data, but priorities may change along the way and our original plan may no longer be appropriate. Don't be afraid to adapt your plan if the bigger picture has changed.

Are our current goals realistic?

Goals which do not have excessive difficulty, can be concretely measured and have a specific timeframe for practice are more motivating than those which seem out of reach (van Leer, 2021) and I agree with this from clinical experience. If the goals you have set are too loose, it will be harder to identify when progress occurs and if they are too ambitious, progress may seem impossible. Tip 19 regarding how to create a therapy plan should help you revise any unrealistic or vaguely specified goals.

How effective is my communication and modelling?

As the quality of our communication contributes to how therapy advice is received (Tips 9 and 10) we should also check that we are explaining and demonstrating the exercises in a way that the client understands, adapting our explanations to account for age, language, and educational differences between clients. You can check that your clients understand what to do by asking them to summarise this for you – if this reveals gaps in understanding, you can provide a reminder of your instructions ensuring this next explanation is more easily accessible. This may mean simplifying your language and/or using written material to supplement verbal explanations.

Am I using high-quality evidence to influence my decision-making?

Speech and language therapists, and indeed all healthcare practitioners, are expected to incorporate the three tenets of evidence-based practice (EBP) – research evidence, clinician experience and client preferences – into their practice (Roddam & Skeat, 2010). Assuming you're providing high-quality instructions and the client is able to process these, we then need to question whether we are using the best available evidence or drawing on outdated practice. Emerging research can consolidate or challenge our existing skills but as learning is career-long, we should continually ask ourselves: is this the most effective way of addressing this difficulty? Contextual and external influences such as service organisation and clinical resources can also limit how EBP is implemented in reality and we may need to think creatively about how we can factor in the limitations whilst still upholding quality intervention.

In the early days of voicework you will have less of your own clinical experience to rely on but you can draw on your supervising therapist's or mentor's wisdom while you develop your personal evidence. Be reassured that your evidence base will come!

Client factors

Does your client understand the current aim of therapy?

If a client is uncertain about the current therapy goal, their practice may become misguided or they may express disappointment that therapy isn't changing their voice if they see this as the exclusive marker of change. However there may be many steps before voice change, including improving vocal health (Tip 21) and developing awareness (Tips 22 and 23), so a gentle reminder may be required as reassurance that non-vocal progress is still being made and is relevant.

Is your client able to understand your communication?

As a bi-directional, shared process, communication not only relies on high-quality information from us but it also relies on the listener (the client) being (a) ready to hear the message and (b) able to understand the message. Burleson's (2009) model of supportive communication, introduced in Tip 4, highlights that clients may not always be open to hearing your advice which can hinder the integration of your guidance.

Is your client completing any home practice?

Progress can be slowed if practice outside clinic sessions is inconsistent or non-existent and this takes us back to Tip 4 regarding behavioural change. Is there any evidence that clients are ready to take action but are finding it difficult to commit to practice on a moment-by-moment basis? What hurdles do they face? What reminder strategies could they use to nudge them to practice or implement the voice care advice you've given? Sometimes it's as simple as a sticky note on the fridge or a digital note on a computer screen as permanently visible reminders but problem solve the challenges with your client so you find a workable solution for them.

Are there any underlying health problems?

If the voice is still not changing as you'd expect despite diligent, accurate practise of appropriate exercises, consider whether there are underlying or undiagnosed medical issues. I remember a client with primary muscle tension dysphonia (MTD) (Tip 27) with no allergy symptoms whose voice was not aided by exercises targeting MTD. Separately their GP prescribed trial antihistamine medications and their voice difficulties quickly resolved, revealing an undiagnosed issue. Silent reflux can also go undiagnosed so you may wish to use a self-rating scale for reflux (Tip 46) and highlight any elevated scores to your client's GP.

When therapy should be postponed or stopped

Whether public funding or an insurance company is funding the sessions, these resources are not limitless. If the challenges preventing attendance or engagement with therapy are short-lived such as a bereavement or temporary ill-health, services may be able to postpone appointments for a few weeks, but if the challenges are longer term or your client does not wish to commit to therapy, you should consider discharge as outlined in Tip 11. In these circumstances, students and newly qualified therapists may either think the client has failed, or indeed has been failed, but they are likely to be discharged with more knowledge about the voice and what SLT can offer than before you met. This understanding should facilitate a reconnection with therapy when circumstances are more conducive to attendance and practice. Some of the wisest decisions we make are the ones where therapy *didn't* happen.

TIP 13 – BEING A CULTURALLY RESPONSIVE THERAPIST

Wrapped around all the other skills in this chapter is cultural responsiveness, our ability to learn from people within our own and other cultures, and relate respectfully with them. Rich cultural diversity in the world is reflected in the diversity of our client backgrounds and RCSLT continues its drive to increase diversity in the profession so the SLT workforce better reflects the membership and those who access our services.

As a starting point, the Cultural Atlas is an excellent online resource to learn more about typical country cultures within categories such as core concepts, religion, greetings, family, communication, and etiquette but remember typical traits are just that – they are not universal. Respecting other cultures isn't exclusive to voicework so this resource is applicable for any placement or rotation. As adapting our responsiveness to others is reliant on self-reflection, try the self-development activity before reading about some specific cultural influences in voicework.

> **SELF-DEVELOPMENT ACTIVITY 13 – REFLECTING ON YOUR INFLUENCES**
>
> Using the Cultural Atlas, look up the country or countries most influential in your life.
>
> - Do these accurately reflect how you experience those cultures?
> - What does this mean for your practice?

The influence of religious beliefs

Ramadan is a month-long period of reflection accompanied by fasting between dawn and sunset for followers of Islam. Aligned with lunar cycles, rather than solar cycles, it occurs around 11 days earlier each year so the period of fasting will be shorter during months with less daylight and longer during months with more daylight. You should be sensitive with your vocal care advice for clients adhering to Ramadan as fluids will not be permitted during the usual waking day. We know that staying well hydrated improves the voice (Tip 21) but for fasting clients with existing dysphonia, the cumulative effect of hypohydration may further increase their vocal effort. Exceptions to fasting during daylight hours are permitted for health reasons. including menstruation, but not all clients choose to follow this exception. An alternative to drinking fluids for systemic hydration is to use 0.9% saline nebulisers or steam inhalations as in self-development activity 6 although some followers also believe the inhalations conflict with Ramadan fasting requirements. Although Büyükatalay et al.'s (2020) research regarding Islamic religious officials does not focus on the influence of Ramadan, this is an interesting paper regarding the communication demands of this professional voice user group and their heightened risk of voice difficulties.

Age-influenced beliefs

The UK National Health Service was hailed a national success in providing free healthcare for everyone, and those alive at the time of its inception in 1948 or born in the years immediately afterwards may believe that "doctor knows best" which extends to "the healthcare professional knows best". Although this belief conflicts with 21st century healthcare principles of promoting shared, collaborative ownership of healthcare plans (Tip 5), its legacy lives on. Some older clients will therefore look to you unquestionably for guidance but we can still encourage client choice by asking "what matters to you?" and identifying meaningful client outcomes as explored in Tip 11.

A characteristic UK stiff upper lip and the belief that we should "grin and bear" troubles means some clients will not approach their general practitioner until a problem is particularly difficult or a kindly family member nudges them to do so. As a result clients may worry they are wasting your time or are not deserving of therapy, and the acknowledgement in the Cultural Atlas that older British people prefer to "mind one's own business" may also mean they do not wish to divulge personal information.

Generational comfort

Experimentation with the voice needs clients to allow themselves to be a little vulnerable – in attempting any task they risk a sound not matching your demonstration, just as you may need to risk a sound that doesn't match the one your supervising therapist or mentor has modelled. In wanting to "get it right", clients may be embarrassed by the attempts that come along the way and van Leer and Connor's (2015) statement in Tip 6 that voice exercises can be plain weird applies here. They may not feel comfortable about lip trills in front of others or someone of an older or younger generation, and discomfort with your exercises may be a barrier to home practice. Make sure you adapt your therapy so your clients feel comfortable with what you are asking of them.

LGBTQIA

Originally LGB, standing for lesbian, gay, and bisexual, the acronym at its longest is now LGBTQQIP2SAA and includes transgender, queer, questioning, intersex, pansexual, two-spirit, androgynous, and asexual communities. Regardless of whether a client discloses their sexuality or their gender identity, we must respect their lifeworld and be non-judgemental regarding others' choices. Gender identities and sexual preferences should not influence the therapy we provide and we should be ready to follow a client's lead in their use of pronouns when they refer to partners or friends whose gender identity goes beyond a he–she dichotomy.

Political cultures

In recent times the UK has experienced a referendum on Scottish independence from the rest of the UK and a referendum on Britain leaving the European Union, alongside other significant changes in international political landscapes. It is difficult to ignore major breaking news within social conversation in sessions but we should be careful in how we navigate this. Some clients with strong political views or affiliations may see an appointment as an opportunity to persuade you of their views but, to be time-efficient, we should avoid lengthy debate, unless of course you can opportunistically exploit the conversation as a voice practise activity!

REFERENCES

Abraham, C. & Sheeran, P. (2005) The Health Belief Model. In Connor, M. & Norman, P. (Ed.) *Predicting health behaviour*. Maidenhead: Open University Press

Alwani, M. M., Campa, K. A., Svenstrup, T. J., Bandali, E. H. & Anthony, B. P. (2021) An Appraisal of Printed Online Education Materials on Spasmodic Dysphonia. *Journal of Voice 35* (4) 659.e1–659.e9 https://doi.org/10.1016/j.jvoice.2019.11.023

Behlau, M., Madazio, G., Pacheco, C., Vaiano, T., Badaró, F. & Barbara, M. (in press) Coaching Strategies for Behavioural Voice Therapy and Training. *Journal of Voice* https://doi.org/10.1016/j.jvoice.2020.12.039

Büyükatalay, Z. C., Gökmen, M. F., Yildrim, S. & Dursun, G. (2020) Voice Disorders in Islamic Religious Officials: Is It Any Different Than Those of the Teachers, Another Well-Known Professional Voice Users? *Journal of Voice 34* (5) 738–742 https://doi.org/10.1016/j.jvoice.2019.02.001

Burleson, B. R. (2009) Understanding the Outcomes of Supportive Conversation: A Dual-process Approach. *Journal of Social and Personal Relationships 26* (1) 21–38 https://doi.org.10.1177/0265407509105519

Burns, K. (2005) *Focus on Solutions. A Health Professional's Guide*. London: Whurr Publishers Ltd.

Doll, E. J., Braden, M. N. & Thibeault, S. L. (2021) Covid-19 and Speech-Language Pathology Clinical Practice of Voice and Upper Airway Disorders. *American Journal of Speech-Language Pathology 30* (1) http://dx.doi.org/10.1044/2020_AJSLP-20-00228

Doruk, C., Enver, N., Çaytemel, B., Azezli, E. & Başaran, B. (2020) Readability, Understandability, and Quality of Online Education Materials for Vocal Fold Nodules. *Journal of Voice 34* (2) 302.e15–302.e20 https://doi.org/10.1016/j.jvoice.2018.08.015

Dueppen, A. J., Bellon-Harn, M. L., Radhakrishnan, N. & Manchaiah, V. (2019) Quality and Readability of English-Language Internet Information for Voice Disorders. *Journal of Voice 33* (3) 290–296 https://doi.org/10.1016/j.jvoice.2017.11.002

Eastwood, C. Madill, C. & McCabe, P. (2015) The Behavioural Treatment of Muscle Tension Voice Disorders: A Systematic Review. *International Journal of Speech-Language Pathology 17* (3) 287–303 https://doi.org/10.3109/17549507.2015.1024169

Ebersole, B., Soni, R. S., Moran, K., Lango, M., Devarajan, K. & Jamal, N. (2017) The Role of Occupational Voice Demand and Patient-Rated Impairment in Predicting Voice Therapy Adherence. *Journal of Voice 32* (3) 325–331 https://doi.org/10.1016/j.jvoice.2017.06.002

Enderby, P., John, A. & Petheram, B. (2006) *Therapy Outcome Measures for the Rehabilitation Professionals: Speech and Language Therapy; Physiotherapy; Occupational Therapy; Rehabilitation Nursing; Hearing Therapists.* Chichester: John Wiley

Gillespie, A. & Gartner-Schmidt, J. (2018) Voice-Specialized Speech-Language Pathologist's Criteria for Discharge from Voice Therapy. *Journal of Voice 32* (3) 332–339 https://doi.org/10.1016/j.jvoice.2017.05.022

Iwarsson, J. (2015) Facilitating Behavioral Learning and Habit Change in Voice Therapy – Theoretic Premises and Practical Strategies. *Logopedics Phoniatrics Vocology 40* (4) 179–186 https://doi.org/10.3109/14015439.2014.936498

Kenny, C. (in press) Dysphonia and Vocal Tract Discomfort While Working From Home During COVID-19. *Journal of Voice* https://doi.org/10.1016/j.jvoice.2020.10.010

Kishbaugh, K.C., Kemper, C. E. & Altman, K. E. (2021) Maintaining Healthy Vocal Use for Teachers During COVID-19 and Beyond. *Journal of Voice* 35 (6) 813–814 https://doi.org/10.1016/j.jvoice.2021.04.001

Knickerbocker, K., Bryan, C. & Ziegler, A. (2021) Phonogenic Voice Problems among Speech-Language Pathologists in Synchronous Telepractice: An Overview and Recommendations. *Seminars in Speech and Language* 42 (1) 73–84 https://doi.org/10.1055/s-0040-1722754

Madill, C., McIlwaine, A., Russell, R., Hodges, N. J. & McCabe, P. (2020) Classifying and Identifying Motor Learning Behaviors in Voice-Therapy Clinician-Client Interactions: A Proposed Motor Learning Classification Framework. *Journal of Voice* 34 (5) 806.e19–806.e31 https://doi.org/10.1016/j.jvoice.2019.03.014

Mannix, K. (2021) *Listen. How to Find the Words for Tender Conversations.* London: William Collins

Marques Torbes, T. M., Zencke da Silva, K., Dalbosco Gadenz, C. & Cassol, M. (2020) Adherence of Patients With Dysphonia to Voice Therapy: Systematic Review. *Journal of Voice* 34 (5) 808.e15–808.e23 https://doi.org/10.1016/j.jvoice.2019.04.008

Roddam, H. & Skeat, J. (2010) *Embedding Evidence-Based Practice in Speech and Language Therapy: International Examples.* Oxford: Wiley-Blackwell

Rubino, M. & Abbott, K. V. (in press) Scoping Review of Voice Therapy Adherence. *Journal of Voice* https://doi.org/10.1016/j.jvoice.2021.09.020

Rumbach, A. F., Dallaston, K. & Hill, A. E. (2021) Student Perceptions of Factors that Influence Clinical Competency in Voice. *International Journal of Speech-Language Pathology* 23 (2) https://doi.org/10.1080/17549507.2020.1737733

Slavych, B. K., Zraick, R. I., Bursac, Z., Tulunay-Ugur, O. & Hadden, K. (2021) An Investigation of the Relationship between Adherence to Voice Therapy for Muscle Tension Dysphonia and Employment, Social Support, and Life

Satisfaction. *Journal of Voice 35* (3) 386–393 https://doi.org/10.1016/j.jvoice.2019.10.015

Sylvestre, A. & Gobeil, S. (2020) The Therapeutic Alliance: A Must for Clinical Practice. *Canadian Journal of Speech-Language Pathology 44* (3) 125–136 Retrieved from: https://cjslpa.ca/files/2020_CJSLPA_Vol_44/No_3/CJSLPA_Vol_44_No_3_2020_1193.pdf

van Leer, E. (2021) Enhancing Adherence to Voice Therapy via Social Cognitive Strategies. *Seminars in Speech and Language 42* (1) 19–31 https://doi.org/10.1055/s-0040-1722755

van Leer, E. & Connor, N. P. (2010) Patient Perceptions of Voice Therapy Adherence. *Journal of Voice 24* (4) 458–469 https://doi.org/10.1016/j.jvoice.2008.12.009.

van Leer, E. & Connor, N. P. (2015) Predicting and Influencing Voice Therapy Adherence Using Social-Cognitive Factors and Mobile Video. *American Journal Speech Language Pathology 24* (2) 164–176 https://doi.org/10.1044/2015_AJSLP-12-0123

van Leer, E., Hapner, E. R. & Connor, N. P. (2008) Transtheoretical Model of Health Behavior Change Applied to Voice Therapy. *Journal of Voice 22* (6) 688–698 https://doi.org/10.1016/j.jvoice.2007.01.011

White, A. C. & Carding, P. (2020) Pre-and Postoperative Voice Therapy for Benign Vocal Fold Lesions: Factors Influencing a Complex Intervention. *Journal of Voice 36* (1) 59–67 https://doi.org/10.1016/j.jvoice.2020.04.004

ADDITIONAL LEARNING RESOURCES

Cultural Atlas www.culturalatlas.sbs.com.au

British Voice Association guidance on remote communication www.britishvoiceassociation.org.uk/voicecare_how-to-maintain-a-heathy-voice-online.htm

RCSLT Telehealth Guidance www.rcslt.org/members/delivering-quality-services/telehealth-guidance/

Chapter 4

ASSESSMENT

Across the five tips in this chapter you are reminded of the components in comprehensive voice assessment and the importance of evaluating the voice from a holistic perspective. We will consider how to evaluate the vocal demands of individual clients, including some staggering measurements of how far the vocal folds travel for professional voice users. After reflecting on the relevance of voice categorisation frameworks to understand the nature of diagnoses, we will consider the fundamental clinical decision of whether we should provide onward therapy.

TIP 14 – AN ASSESSMENT CHECKLIST

Voice assessment begins from the moment you say hello to your client. Whether social conversation occurs during the walk from the waiting area to a therapy room or at the start of an online therapy session, this isn't just about connecting with the client – you're using this as an early opportunity to evaluate their voice in spontaneous conversation. Student SLTs may be tempted to include a specific activity in your session plan to build rapport with your clients but, in reality, a short, friendly conversation is sufficient to convey a positive first impression with the added bonus of providing valuable data.

As whole sections of academic textbooks are devoted to the assessment process, I will not repeat everything here though I guide you to Stachler et al. (2018) for comprehensive, multidisciplinary recommendations including some helpful questions to use in your initial appointment. Martin (2021) neatly summarises relevant case history information with rationale and she also provides a case history template. Finally, Shewell's (2009) eight parameters within her Voice Skills Perceptual Profile provide a structure within which you can explore specific aspects of the voice to guide intervention.

Ensuring comprehensiveness

High-quality, holistic information should cover all aspects of the client's well-being including the history of the problem, their social network, their medical care, their emotional and psychological health, and the impact of their voice difficulties. In voicework it is difficult, and unwise, to make a mind–body distinction, for what we are experiencing psychologically and emotionally is often mirrored physically. I view initial sessions as a puzzle in which I go on a hunt for all the relevant information which, pieced together, allows me to move nearer to the root cause of the difficulty and translate this into layperson's terms for the client, and I encourage you to approach data gathering with similar curiosity.

In the early stages of your development, it may be challenging to make observations and conversation simultaneously, but choose an aspect, or a couple of aspects, of voice assessment to focus on for the day and then a couple of different ones the following day, and you'll soon build up your skills.

> **SELF-DEVELOPMENT ACTIVITY 14 – PRACTISING ASSESSMENT**
>
> If you have not carried out voice assessment recently, it is time well spent to practise this. Find a willing housemate, friend, or family member and test out your questions so the first time you hear yourself explain an activity is not in clinic. If you are using a session planning template as a student I strongly encourage you to include scripts for each activity.
>
> After you've practised, ask yourself:
>
> - What have I learnt from practising case history gathering and assessment?
> - What do I need to do now to develop my confidence and/or skills?

Do I know what the vocal folds look like?

Prior to assessment you should be familiar with the vocal fold appearances associated with the different diagnoses. The client's voice quality you hear may sound like Reinke's oedema or presbyphonia, but only through endoscopic evaluation of the larynx (EEL) will a diagnosis be confirmed. My ENT colleagues also recommend you know what normal vocal folds look like – in a voice clinic you may often see abnormal functioning or appearance but you should also be able to recognise a healthy, fully functioning larynx.

What can be heard on assessment?

Information regarding the problem and client's lifeworld will be supplemented by acoustic-perceptual data and your department may have a specific recording form for this.

Acoustic analysis

Conventional measures include jitter (frequency perturbation), shimmer (amplitude perturbation), and harmonic-to-noise ratio, but updated Cepstral software now complements this more traditional acoustic evaluation. While conventional measures and Cepstral Peak Prominence (CPP) both have value (Hassan et al., 2021), not all SLT clinics have access to the necessary software for acoustic evaluation so we also need an alternative, readily accessible assessment tool for perceptual analysis: our ears.

Perceptual analysis

As a "portable, in-your-pocket" means of perceptual evaluation, the GRBAS scale asks therapists to rate the perceived deviation from a normal voice across five items: the overall grade (G), roughness (R), breathiness (B), asthenia (A) (weakness), and strain (S). The scale's four points range from 0–3, where 0 reflects no deviation from a normal voice, 1 reflects mild deviation, 2 is moderate deviation, and a score of 3 means there is severe deviation from normal voice production. Most often your voice and mine will have a rating of $G_0 R_0 B_0 A_0 S_0$ unless we have a cold or have been overusing our voices, and in Chapter 6 you will learn which of these parameters change with the different voice diagnoses. Dejonckere et al. (1996) later extended the scale with an instability rating to reflect fluctuations in voice quality, making it GRBASI. To develop your rating skills in listening to everyday voices and using this scale, return to Tip 3 and try self-development activity 7.

The GRBAS scale isn't just reserved for initial assessment though, and you should have this in mind in any session. Is this the extent of difficulty you were expecting based on the referral letter or any previous contact with your client? Can you hear any difference as clients start using their voice differently? Can you hear differences between specific practice and spontaneous conversation? Maybe it doesn't sound disordered at all!

In a final therapy session, and alongside discussion of self-rating scores, I share my GRBAS ratings with clients as additional evidence of change (or not as the case may be) and explain what each of the items mean. I may also share ratings when there is significant change during the therapy process as this information can be motivating for clients to continue practice.

An alternative audio-perceptual scale is the Consensus Auditory-Perceptual Evaluation of Voice (CAPE-V) (Zraick et al., 2011). Like GRBAS, the CAPE-V also has an overall severity rating and ratings for roughness, breathiness, and strain, but replaces asthenia with loudness and, unlike GRBAS, includes a pitch evaluation, specific tasks to gather data, and uses a continuous scale to reflect the continuum of voices.

Client-led perceptual evaluation occurs outside of a clinic environment and some clients may bring mobile phone recordings for you to hear between-session practice. Although accurate acoustic analysis using mobile phone technology is still under development (Jannetts et al., 2019; Petrizzo & Popolo, 2021), these at-home recordings should be sufficient for a broad idea of between-appointment progress between appointments.

Client self-ratings

Combining our evaluation of a client's voice with their own perception provides a more rounded picture and can be particularly informative where our judgement does not match theirs. Inviting client report of the difficulties upholds the spirit of collaborative working (Tip 5) and will also influence the decision to offer therapy or not (Tip 19).

Alongside a verbal description of their experiences, client opinion is typically gathered via self-assessment scales. The

30-item Voice Handicap Index (VHI) (Jacobsen et al., 1997) covers functional, physical, and emotional aspects of the voice and there is the shorter, similarly valid 10-item scale (Rosen et al., 2004). The Vocal Tract Discomfort Scale (VTDS) (Mathieson et al., 2009) focuses on symptoms and sensations reflecting discomfort and is validated in several languages including Spanish (Argentina), Portuguese (Brazil), German, Polish, Persian, Turkish, Italian, Korean, and Arabic. Finally, the Voice-Related Quality of Life (V-RQOL) (Hogikyan & Sethuraman, 1999) focuses on how voice difficulties impact on day-to-day activities. The VTDS is in Appendix 1.

In being time and context dependent, self-rating scales are susceptible to external influences, so pay attention when a client complains about not being able to get a car parking space for their appointment and is then immediately asked to rate their voice! Greater vocal demands may also contribute to a greater perception of impairment (Ebersole et al., 2017) and clients experiencing dysphonia for longer may have lower self-rating scores than those whose difficulties are more recent (Behrman et al., 2004). This doesn't mean that all clients with recent-onset difficulties have over-inflated scores, or that all clients with longstanding difficulties underestimate the impairment, but the numerical data should be supplemented by discussion with the client. You could say: *"I see you've rated the actual problem fairly low on this scale but the impact of that seems more significant. Can you tell me more about that?"* Alternatively, you might comment: *"You've rated your actual voice difficulties as being really quite significant here but they don't seem to be having much impact on you day-to-day. Would that be right?"*

SELF-DEVELOPMENT ACTIVITY 15 – RATING YOUR OWN VOICE

Complete either of the self-rating assessments in Appendix 1, also available for download from www.routledge.com/cw/speechmark, so you have experience

> of reflecting on your voice using a structured tool, remembering that it can be difficult to reach an absolute 0 on self-rating assessments due to natural variation in our voices across the day or other health symptoms, such as reflux or post-nasal drip.

Now you know what data you need, use the checklist below when planning your sessions to ensure you have accounted for all sources of data.

Have I already gathered information, or have planned to gather information, about:	
- what the vocal folds look like and how they are functioning?	❑
- the background to the client's difficulties, their work, social, medical and psychological context?	❑
- how the voice sounds on a range of assessment tasks?	❑
- the wider picture of the client's body	❑
- the client's opinion about their voice difficulties	❑

TIP 15 – JUDGING AMOUNT OF VOICE USE

In gathering data about what your clients use their voice for, you will start to have a sense of whether they are voice overdoers or underdoers (Bastian & Thomas, 2016) but how do we judge whether there is too much or too little voice use?

Understanding the terminology

Within the literature you will come across terms such as "vocal load", "vocal demand", "vocal effort", and "vocal fatigue" with some used interchangeably or without agreed definition. Vocal load and vocal loading are both used to refer to vocal use which contributes to an excessive vocal load, the process by which the voice is overloaded or the additional demand we deliberately create to extend voice skills, such as asking the client to practise against background noise or developing pitch flexibility and loudness capabilities (Hunter et al., 2020). Vocal fatigue is also variably defined in research but broadly describes muscle fatigue leading to bodily tension, reduced vocal flexibility, a weaker voice, and increasing symptoms across the day. To reduce confusion going forward, Hunter et al. (2020) propose two new terms of *vocal demand* – the vocal requirements for any given situation – and *vocal demand response* as the way by which a speaker attempts to meet the vocal demand through integrating their individual physiology, their perception of environmental acoustics, previous vocal knowledge and training, and their in-the-moment social and emotional state. Appreciating the heterogeneity in vocal demand responses starts to reveal why some of our clients run in to trouble where colleagues doing the same job do not.

Within Hunter et al.'s proposition of vocal demand, we can also incorporate vocal fold exposure to vibration which can be calculated from phonation time, fundamental frequency, and vocal intensity. It is summarised by Assad et al. (2017) as comprising:

- the amount of **time** vocal folds are vibrating
- the number of **vibratory cycles** over a given time

- the **distance** travelled by the vocal folds during their vibration, which is influenced by amplitude
- the amount of **heat** produced in the vocal folds

Gathering data about amount of voice use

Clinicians "on the ground" are unlikely have access to the research vocal dosimeters to measure vocal fold exposure to vibration but broad evaluation is still possible by asking our clients:

- how long do you use your voice use (a) at any one time and (b) across the day? Isolated periods of consistent voice use during an hour-long business pitch result in a different time dose from sustained voice use across the day in a teaching environment.
- what pitch changes do you need across different conversations or within specific situations? A primary school teacher may use a variety of character voices at story time which challenge pitch flexibility or a performer may have a musical theatre repertoire which stretches their pitch range. Higher pitches increase the number of vibratory cycles.
- how loud does your voice need to be? What noise do you compete with and for how long? Our observations of the client's conversational voice may hint at habitual amplitude levels, as well as those reported in work or social environments, and a gauge of amplitude contributes to an evaluation of distance and heat doses.

The role of therapy in managing voice use

Using vocal demand, vocal demand response, and vocal fold exposure to vibration as a context, you should be able to identify where the challenges in amount of voice use lie. You will meet very talkative clients who may speak loudly, describe themselves as the "life and soul of the party", and if you are meeting them in-person you might even hear them talking to everyone in the waiting room – these are the voice overdoers.

We are not aiming to change exuberant, bubbly personalities but some of our clients may need to think about using their voice more conservatively.

There have been some fascinating calculations of the number of metres vocal folds vibrate in professional voice users including 7000 m (almost four miles) for music teachers and 3688 m for classroom elementary (primary) teachers *each day* (Morrow & Connor, 2011), between 2500–3000 m for call centre workers (Cantarella et al., 2014), and around 2500 m for indoor cycling instructors in just an hour (Allison et al., 2020). It is these figures which may mean your clients take notice when you encourage them to consider voice conservation! Where the time dose is increased due to prolonged use, you will likely consider a recommendation of short periods of voice rest. Where the number of oscillatory cycles is high with greater pitch variation, you may identify where this can be reduced (Tip 41 regarding educators considers how pitch can be modified), remembering that many singers have specific requirements regarding the pitch range they are to use. Where distance and heat doses are elevated due to projection of the voice, a microphone can decrease some of the vocal intensity.

You will also meet clients who use their voice far less or speak quietly, and they are considered the voice underdoers. In this case we might wish to increase some aspects of vocal dose and how to do this is described in Tip 35. As with any continuum, of course, there will also be clients for whom overuse or underuse are not factors influencing the voice but as a general rule we should all factor in some voice rest during the day.

TIP 16 – ASSESSMENT AS EXPERIMENTATION

Alongside the required assessment data, your initial session is also an opportunity for experimentation to gauge potential therapeutic stimulability and vocal variability.

Experimentation to find the solution

Within early conversation and assessment tasks you may notice variability in the client's voice which can be recorded on the instability parameter of GRBASI (Dejonckere et al., 1996). Although an unstable voice sounds undesirable, variability is evidence that easier or more effective phonation is possible and the presenting difficulty is not fully embedded. Highlighting this can offer reassurance to our clients and, if time permits in an assessment session, you can explore the more effective phonation to introduce and reinforce early vocal control. In adopting solution-focused thinking, if we can identify what is working well in the voice, can our client's do more of it?

Experimentation to test stimulability

Overlapping with variability, early vocal experimentation gauges how responsive the client's voice may be in onward therapy. For example, if your client's voice is of normal quality but quiet on perceptual assessment, ask them to try the tasks with greater intensity to evaluate how they think they improve their attempt without your modelling. A louder attempt with no strain quickly confirms scope for improved projection and even a louder attempt accompanied by strain provides useful information about aspects of therapy you may wish to address.

For clients whose voice problem appears to be influenced, at least in part, by muscle tension I often include lip trills at the end of my standard assessment activities. This exercise is both a good tension reducer (Tip 25) and tension identifier. This can be done with and without phonation, and tension emerging in the phonated version may allude to vocal tension in conversation. If spontaneous trills are difficult clients may be aided by pretending to be cold (saying "brr" with their arms wrapped round them) or by placing their forefingers either side of their lips in a vertical position as they attempt the trill. Where these are part of your assessment you're unlikely to have time to provide the same level of support as in a dedicated therapy session so present each trial as gentle experimentation to reduce any pressure to succeed at therapy tasks during your first meeting.

When asking clients to experiment in this way I listen out for, and highlight, any subtle changes in the voice which suggest continued adaptation is possible – it is often important for clients to leave the first appointment with a belief there is scope for a positive outcome from therapy. Even if brief experimentation does not bring improved vocal experiences, it doesn't mean the voice will never change and an intrigued client may continue to practise your task at home spontaneously with later audible benefit.

TIP 17 – SUMMARISING YOUR FINDINGS: WHAT'S IN A LABEL?

During our training we learn about the different disorders of communication, eating, drinking, and swallowing, using the typical symptoms of each disorder to label what we are seeing or hearing and plan therapy. A longstanding approach to voice disorder classification is to describe them as *organic* or *non-organic*, which are now explained.

Organic disorders

Here, a change in the body's structure or physiology causes the dysphonia, as in vocal fold nodules or the laryngeal irritation caused by gastro-oesophageal reflux. Historically, the nerve damage in a vocal fold palsy has also been considered organic though Hacki et al. (2022) find this a confusing distinction in that dysphonia caused by neural interruption is related to the brain system rather than an organ.

Non-organic disorders

In non-organic disorders there is a malfunction of the voice, which contributes to the alternative term of "functional difficulties", but this is not to be confused with functional neurological disorder (FND) in which distress interrupts neurological pathways and is characterised by inconsistent communication and swallowing symptoms with no determined cause for the difficulties. Hacki et al. (2022) consider functional dysphonia to be a rather vague term and see non-organic as a statement only of what the dysphonia is not caused by. As an alternative they propose "malregulative dysphonia" to reflect a faulty voice production system without an organic cause. They also argue that "phonation disorder" should replace "voice disorder" as dysphonia is not always the most significant symptom and certainly vocal tract discomfort or fatigue may be more dominant. As the emergence of new terms coincides with the development of this book, it is not clear whether they will be picked up by the voice community, so watch this space!

Returning to more common terminology, functional difficulties are separated into those primarily caused by muscle tension and ineffective use of the muscles (muscle tension dysphonia), and those which are considered to be caused by emotional distress (psychogenic dysphonia) which are further explored in Tips 27 and 28 respectively. Figure 5 clarifies this distinction.

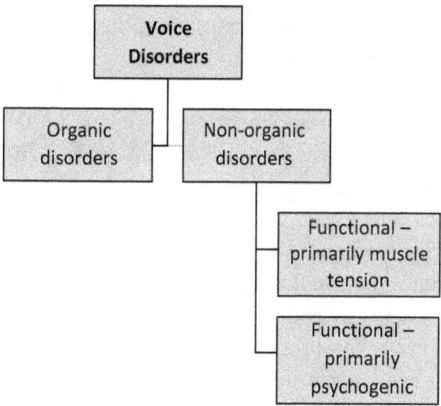

Figure 5 Classification of voice disorders

Viewing disorders differently

Although this longstanding classification helps us identify whether there is a medical, functional, or psychogenic cause for the difficulties, it assumes voice difficulties can be tidied into neat little boxes which definitely isn't the case. The classification doesn't take account of the multifactorial nature of voice difficulties and the relationship between the different influencing factors. For instance, in the classification system above, a client with age-related physiological changes would be considered to present with an organic voice disorder but where the difficulties lead to maladaptive voice production in a bid to overcome the problem, there is also a behavioural, or non-organic, element.

Rather than compartmentalising voice difficulties, the voice can be viewed as a kaleidoscope of influencing factors, using the 4P model to tease out how and when the different factors make their effect known. This model comprises unhelpful Predisposing, Precipitating, and Perpetuating factors, and more helpfully, Protective factors. Predisposing factors, which place a client at greater risk of developing dysphonia could include a diagnosis of asthma and/or working as a teacher. A precipitating factor which results in the current dysphonia may be a winter cold but the perpetuating factor, which keeps the problem going, is the whispering the client used when they lost their voice. Positively, a protective factor might be that the client already drinks plenty of water to stay hydrated. Thinking back to the information you gather in your initial case history and initial assessment (Tip 14), each of these predisposing, precipitating, perpetuating, and protective factors could relate to the client's physical health (including ENT diagnosis), their mental well-being, their environment (including their job), their vocal health, and how they produce voice. What a melting pot of possible influences there can be.

As well as aiding therapy planning, the 4P model also supports clients to understand how their difficulties have evolved, have realistic expectations about therapy, increase the amount of responsibility they take on for their voice, and encourage them to practise specific exercises. But how do we distil the many possible factors into a way clients can follow?

Written summaries can be helpful, both as a permanent reference for the client and as a bonus memory aid for us to ensure we cover everything in our explanations. Figure 6 shows an example of a 4P summary and a blank copy is in Appendix 2, also available for download from www.routledge.com/cw/speechmark, if you wish to use this template with your clients. When working in-person, clients can add their own written notes as you discuss the factors but it's also possible to use this during remote therapy via shared screens and emailing copies of the information to clients after the session.

What is contributing to my voice difficulties?

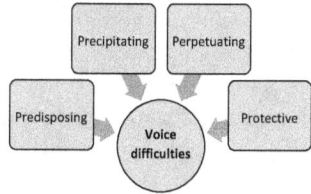

- Predisposing – what increases my risk of having voice problems?
- Precipitating – what has caused this episode of voice difficulties?
- Perpetuating – what is keeping the voice difficulties going?
- Protective – what can help me reduce the voice difficulties or my risk of voice difficulties?

	Predisposing	Precipitating	Perpetuating	Protective
My physical health	Asthma	Winter cold with a week's voice loss		
My mental health			Work can be stressful	Practice yoga and mindfulness
My environment	Being a teacher. Open-plan school		More voice use while covering for colleague	
My vocal care	Trying to sing above noise when clubbing		New throat clearing	Drink plenty of water
My voice production style	Can speak quickly, not always pausing for breath		Newly added strain to compensate for the hoarseness	Occasionally use neck stretches at work

Figure 6 Sample summary of the 4P influencing factors for a client

TIP 18 – TO PLAN THERAPY OR NOT?

With sufficient data, in both its amount and its quality, you will be able to decide what support SLT can offer and whether intervention is appropriate. Simply put, your choices are discharging with advice, referring the client onwards to other services, or providing a block of therapy with or without a concomitant onward referral. Let's take a look at these possible decisions, including the reasons why you may discharge a client without therapy.

Discharge with advice regarding voice care if difficulties have resolved

Do you remember my final university exam client mentioned in the Introduction? The gap between clients attending for laryngeal assessment and their initial SLT appointment may allow difficulties to resolve so do not be surprised (like I was!) if a client reports the problem no longer exists. They may have attended their appointment out of sense of duty or because they don't want to miss out on relevant information from you. If the precipitating factors leading to the recent episode of dysphonia no longer exist, there are no ongoing factors suggesting the client continues to be at risk, and they have no vocal concerns, you can comfortably discharge a client after providing voice care advice so they are generally aware of the importance of vocal health.

Do check with your client that they are happy with the discharge – even if the difficulties no longer exist, a quick discharge may be unexpected but sharing your clinical rationale will demonstrate that your decision is well-considered. You could say: *"I can hear your voice is normal in conversation and the [insert what caused the difficulty] has now resolved. Many voice difficulties can be temporary and I'm sure you're pleased these have now gone. Other than generally looking after your voice as we discussed, there is nothing more we need to do together. What do you think?"*

Discharge with advice regarding voice care if the client does not wish to attend

Although a referral to SLT has been initiated, that in itself doesn't oblige a client to attend therapy. When offering intervention, explain what aspect of the voice you would like to address, an overview of how you intend to reach the goals and what you hope therapy will achieve. With this information clients can make an informed decision about their care, and this shared ownership of treatment decisions is encouraged in the UK. Incorporating what you know from Tip 4 regarding behavioural change and Tip 5 regarding collaborative working, it is therefore an entirely valid course of action to discharge someone if they do not wish to attend and you have discussed this with them.

Discharge with advice regarding voice care if the client would like to attend but is unable to commit to ongoing therapy at present

Ideally, the client's personal circumstances will create space for therapy but changes in their lifeworld, including family commitments, health problems or bereavements can interrupt regular attendance. Although this may be disappointing for you and your client if you can both see the value in SLT attendance, we are not always able to prevent the impact of life realities. Depending on your service organisation, it may be possible for clients to resume therapy once circumstances settle if these are predicted to be temporary.

Discharge with onward referral

During your data-gathering conversations clients may talk extensively about wider health ailments or life frustrations with you which, although they might have some relevance for our work, may also be an indication of other priorities or greater challenges than the voice. For some clients, the most helpful service may not be SLT – more beneficial services may already be known to the client if they are attending other clinics, such as a respiratory clinic for chronic obstructive pulmonary disease (most usually referred to as COPD), or they may be new services such as a smoking cessation team or counselling. If you are able to refer directly to other services, do acknowledge this in your discharge report so the GP and referring agent are clear about your rationale for not providing SLT input. If you are not able to refer directly elsewhere you can include a professional request for the GP to do this in your correspondence.

Provide a block of therapy +/- onward referral

Although this tip has been dominated by the reasons for discharge post-assessment, for many clients you will plan a block of therapy and work with voice difficulties of varying degrees of impairment and impact.

The referral information can help us to hypothesise at an early stage which clients may benefit from, and will be interested in, further therapy, but don't hold your assumptions too closely. Education from you about what is possible may just persuade some clients to attend where they otherwise had no intention to do so. Use self-development activity 16 below to start thinking about who you might predict will attend for therapy and why.

> **SELF-DEVELOPMENT ACTIVITY 16 – EARLY PREDICTIONS OF CLIENT ATTENDANCE**
>
> Read these hypothetical referrals and, bearing in mind that subsequent data may change your decision,
>
> a) what do you see as the impact for each client?
> b) do you think you might provide therapy?
>
> Suggested answers are in the self-development activities online.

GP referral to ENT 1
Mrs. A attended today with concerns about increasing difficulties singing in Church. She was widowed recently and her connection with her Church network has been a valuable support during difficult times, so she is finding it particularly upsetting to struggle to sing.

GP referral to ENT 2
Mr. B has requested a referral to ENT as he is concerned about intermittent changes to his voice. A close relative passed away a year ago from throat cancer and he is concerned he has the same issue, despite there being no red flags for cancer. He does not smoke, exercises regularly, and denies stress in his job as a public speaker. There is a background of anxiety which Mr. Y tries to address through meditation.

ENT referral for SLT assessment 1
Mr. X was seen in the clinic today and flexible nasoendoscopy revealed extensive Reinke's oedema. As a salesman he is reliant on his voice for work and acknowledges that customers frequently enquire if he has a sore throat which he finds frustrating. He is not concerned about the quality of his voice when with his friends. I have discussed the importance of stopping smoking with him but he is reluctant to do so as he tells me he uses it as a coping mechanism for work stress. I would be grateful if you could see him for an initial assessment and continue the discussion regarding smoking cessation with him.

> ENT referral for SLT assessment 2
> *Ms. Y attended the clinic and videostroboscopy revealed small, soft vocal fold nodules. She is in her final year of studying French and is hoping to start teacher training next year. She is concerned that her voice will prevent her from being successful in her interview or indeed, prevent her from passing her teaching placements. She works in a bar three nights a week with live music playing on two of these evenings. She acknowledges her voice tires by the end of these evenings but has recovered by Monday when she uses her voice in tutorials. I would be grateful if you could see and advise.*

REFERENCES

Allison, L. H., Sandage, M. J., & Weaver, A. J. (2020) Vocal Dose for Rhythm-Based Indoor Cycling Instructors With and Without Amplification. *Journal of Voice* 34 (6) 963.e23–963.e31 https://doi.org/10.1016/j.jvoice.2019.05.010

Assad, J. P., de castro Magalhães, Santos, J. N. & Gama, A. C. C. (2017) Vocal Dose: An Integrative Literature Review. *Speech, Language, Hearing Sciences and Education Journal* 19 (3) 429–438 https://doi.org/10.1590/1982-021620171932617

Bastian, R. W. & Thomas, J. P. (2016) Do Talkativeness and Vocal Loudness Correlate With Laryngeal Pathology? A Study of the Vocal Overdoer/Underdoer Continuum. *Journal of Voice* 30 (5) 557–562 https://doi.org/10.1016/j.jvoice.2015.06.012

Behrman, A., Sulica, L. & He, T. (2004) Factors Predicting Patient Perception of Dysphonia Caused by Benign Vocal Fold Lesions. *The Laryngoscope* 114 1693–1700

Cantarella, G., Iofrida, E., Boria, P., Giordana, S., Binatti, O., Pignatoro, L., Manfredim C., Forti, S. & Dejonckere, P. (2014) Ambulatory Phonation Monitoring in a Sample of 92 Call Center Operators. *Journal of Voice 28* (3) 393.e1–393.e6 https://doi.org/10.1016/j.j.voice.2013.10.002

Dejonckere, P. H., Remacle, M., Fresnel-Elbaz, E., Woisard, V., Crevier-Buchman, L. & Millet, B. (1996) Differentiated Perceptual Evaluation of Pathological Voice Quality: Reliability and Correlations with Acoustic Measurements. *Revue de laryngologie – otologie – rhinologie 117* (3) 219–224

Ebersole, B., Soni, R. S., Moran, K., Lango, M. & Devarajan, K. (2017) The Influence of Occupation on Self-perceived Vocal Problems in Patients With Voice Complaints. *Journal of Voice 32* (6) 673–680 https://doi.org/10.1016/j.jvoice.2017.08.028

Hacki, T., Moerman, M. & Rubin. J. S. (2022) 'Malregulative' Rather Than 'Functional' Dysphonia: A New Etiological Terminology Framework for Phonation Disorders – A Position Paper by the Union of European Phoniatricians (UEP). *Journal of Voice 36* (1) 50–53 https://doi.org/10.1016/j.jvoice.2020.04.032

Hassan, E. M., Hady, A. F. A., Shohdi, S, S., Eldessouky, H. M. & Din, M. H. B. (2021) Assessment of Dysphonia: Cepstral Analysis Versus Conventional Acoustic Analysis. *Logopedics Phoniatrics Vocology 46* (3) 99–109 https://doi.org/10.1080/14015439.2020.1767202

Hogikyan, N. D. & Sethuraman, G. (1999) Validation of an Instrument to Measure Voice-Related Quality of Life (V-RQOL). *Journal of Voice 13* (4) 557–569 https://doi.org/10.1016/So892-1997(99)80010-1

Hunter, E. J., Cantor-Cutiva, L. C., van Leer, E., Mersbergen, M., Nanjundeswaran, C. D., Bottalico, P., Sandage, M. J. & Whitling, S. (2020) Towards a Consensus Description of Vocal Effort, Vocal Load, Vocal Loading, and Vocal Fatigue. *Journal of Speech, Language and Hearing Research 63* (2) 509–532 https://doi.org/10.1044/2019_JSLHR-19-00057

Jacobsen, B. H., Johnson, A., Grywalski, C., Silbergleit, A., Jacobsen, G. (1997) The Voice Handicap Index (VHI) Development and Validation. *American Journal of Speech-Language Pathology 6* (3) 66–70 https://doi.org/10.1044/1058-0360.0603.66

Jannetts, S., Schaeffler, F., Beck, J. & Cowen, S. (2019) Assessing Voice Health Using Smartphones: Bias and Random Error of Acoustic Voice Parameters Captured by Different Smartphone Types. *International Journal of Language & Communication Disorders 54* (2) 292–305 https://doi.org.10.1111/1460-6984.1257

Martin, S. (2021) *Working With Voice Disorders. Theory and Practice.* (3rd Ed.) Abingdon: Routledge

Mathieson, L, Hirani, S. P., Epstein, R., Baken, R. J., Wood, G. & Rubin, J. S. (2009) Laryngeal Manual Therapy: A Preliminary Study to Examine Its Treatment Effects in the Management of Muscle Tension Dysphonia. *Journal of Voice 23* (3) 353–366 https://doi.org.10.1016/j.jvoice.2007.10.002

Morrow, S. L. & Connor, N. P. (2011) Comparison Voice-Use Profiles Between Elementary Classroom and Music Teachers. *Journal of Voice 25* (3) 367–372 https://doi.org/10.1016/j.jvoice.2009.11.006

Petrizzo, D. & Popolo, P. S. (2021) Smartphone Use in Clinical Voice Recording and Acoustic Analysis: A Literature Review. *Journal of Voice 35* (3) 499.e23–499.e28 https://doi.org/10.1016/j.jvoice.2019.10.006

Rosen, C. A., Lee, A. S., Osborne, J., Zullo, T. & Murry, T. (2004) Development and Validation of the Voice Handicap Index-10. *Laryngoscope 114* 9 1549–1556 https://doi.org/10.1097/00005537-200409000-00009

Shewell, C. (2009) *Voice Work. Art and Science in Changing Voices.* Chichester: Wiley-Blackwell

Stachler, R. J., Francis, D. O., Schwartz, S. R., Damask, C. C., Digoy, G. P., Krouse, H. J., McCoy, S. J., Ouellette, D. R., Patel, R. R., Reavis, C. W., Smith, L. J., Smith, M., Strode, S. W., Woo, P. & Nnacheta, L. C. (2018) Clinical Practice Guideline: Hoarseness (Dysphonia) (Update)

Otolaryngology-Head and Neck Surgery (158) (1_suppl) 1–42 https://doi.org/10.1177/0194599817751030

Zraick, R. I., Kempster, G. B., Connor, N. P., Thibeault, S., Klaben, B. K., Bursac, Z., Thrush, C. R. & Glaze, L. E. (2011) Establishing Validity of the Consensus Auditory-Perceptual Evaluation of Voice (CAPE-V) *American Journal of Speech-Language Pathology 20* (1) 14–22 https://dx.doi.org/10.1044/1058-0360(2010/09-0105)

Chapter 5

MANAGEMENT

In this chapter we move from a systematic, but flexible, assessment process to the craft of planning therapy which is both evidence-based and tailored to the needs of the individual clients. The eight tips presented in this chapter include the first steps in creating a management plan, using awareness to heighten your client's learning about their voice and expanding their evaluation beyond what they hear. Consideration is given to breathwork and semi-occluded vocal tract therapy as frequently cited aspects of therapy, and discussion of how voice skills can be generalised using top-down or bottom-up approaches concludes the chapter.

TIP 19 - CREATING A THERAPY PLAN

You've gathered the relevant information, you and your client agree that therapy would be beneficial so now what do you do? How do you know which techniques and practice activities will be right to meet the two key intervention goals of *reducing the severity of the voice problem* where possible and *reducing the resultant impact* on work, personal life, and overall well-being (Ebersole et al., 2017)?

Considering the impairment

The presence of impairment may well be reflected by an audible change in voice quality but this is not true for all clients as strain, fatigue, or vocal tract discomfort are also valid voice symptoms. Even if we can't hear the impairment, if a client says they have a problem and can sense this, we trust that they have a problem.

In the early days of your voicework, a structure such as Shewell's Voice Skills Framework (2009) can be a helpful aid to planning. Start at the top of the framework, which hierarchically considers the body, breath, channel, phonation, resonance, pitch, loudness, and articulation, and use the structure to decide which parameters are the greatest priority for therapy. If there is no obvious body tension, for example, we do not need to address this subsystem, but if there is audible, visible, or felt tension in the vocal tract, working at the level of the channel becomes a clearer focus.

Data evaluation may consider each parameter individually in order to identify problematic aspects but when planning your therapy do return to whole-system thinking so you can exploit the opportunities to address multiple subsystems with one exercise (Madill et al., 2021). Although starting at the top of a framework allows us to evaluate each subsystem systematically, we don't have to treat each subsystem discretely and difficulties are often multifactorial so it is usually not helpful to focus on individual components exclusively (Martin, 2021). For instance, addressing laryngeal constriction may simultaneously reinforce a low-placed breath which means both channel and breath subsystems are strengthened with one deconstriction exercise.

Considering the impact

I've lost count of the number of times clients have commented "I appreciate your time as you must have plenty of people to see who are worse than me". My response always acknowledges the impact of the voice problem as justification for therapy – if dysphonia is hindering interaction with others, influencing life choices, or reducing quality of life, it is right that we offer support. Mild hoarseness may have little impact on someone who does not rely on their voice for their job but it may be the difference between performing and cancelling a high-profile gig for an elite performer. Because of this we can never ignore the impact, which is why it is crucial to enquire about it in our initial appointment (Tip 14).

Where the impact is functional, your plan to address the specific impairment should bring a secondary gain of reducing the impact of the problem. Greater vocal stamina and improved vocal health, for instance, are positive changes in themselves but there is greater functional impact if the client is now able to fulfil their working responsibilities with greater ease, reducing the risk of voice-related sick leave and increasing their emotional well-being. Some clients will spontaneously comment on lessening negative impact, whilst others will benefit from more direct questioning about whether the functional impact is changing alongside voice improvement.

Where the impact of the voice difficulties is emotional, your knowledge regarding tender conversations (Tip 7) will allow you to support and listen to your client. Not all of our therapy will change the underlying problem – spasmodic dysphonia is incurable (Tip 34), laryngeal papillomas may recur (Tip 37), and a vocal fold palsy may not fully resolve (Tip 32), or uncontrollable life stressors have a continuing impact on the body so we need to walk alongside our client as they adjust to new diagnoses or long-term difficulties. An SLT appointment in which there is no practice of exercises but authentic listening from you which enables your client to explore the emotional impact is absolutely valid if that's what's most useful for that client. We don't always have to be making noises in therapy!

Finally, where there is occupational impact, liaison with the client's employer or Access to Work may be required and Tip 49 guides you more specifically with this.

Progressing your plan

Once you've considered how you can address the impairment and impact, it's time to put your plan into action. If you have a session planning template as a student or recent graduate (or as a more qualified therapist who can pinch one of your student's templates) use these to think about your overall aim for this block of therapy and then break down that aim to smaller goals which guide you towards individual activities and the focus for each appointment.

To assist with your planning, think about what you want your client to be able to do or know that they do not currently do or know, as introduced in Tip 11 regarding outcomes, and you can apply this principle to one session or across the whole block of therapy. Short- and long-term goals can be aligned with the SMART acronym in being Specific, Measurable, Achievable, Relevant, and Time-bound, and as with other collaborative decisions (Tip 5), you and your client should agree the goals together.

Adding flair

In Tip 11 possible therapy outcomes included the client's voice returning to a level of function which allows them to participate in a variety of situations, and that may be the point at which therapy is concluded. For other clients, attending voice therapy becomes an opportunity to explore the full scope of the voice for even greater efficiency which Shewell (2009) labels as "extension skills". A teacher returning to work after resolution of nodules, for example, doesn't just need a voice which has a clear quality – they need a voice with stamina and one which captures the interest of their students and projects across a range of educational spaces. A parent of young children with resolved aphonia after laryngitis doesn't just need their voice for conversations about school or nursery – they need it to call the family for dinner and safely animate the characters in bedtime story books. A comedian with a longstanding history of vocal fatigue, exacerbated by recent psychogenic dysphonia from a sudden bereavement and financial stress, doesn't just need a voice which lasts during phone conversations with their agent – they need a voice which is expressive and entertaining for the stage. Can you see how intervention may go beyond simply achieving a normal voice quality for your clients? By considering the unique impact of the difficulty for the client, frequently returning to what matters to them, and considering the level of voice expertise required, you will be able to decide how far voice exploration will continue for your clients. Shewell (2009) and Martin (2021) are good sources of therapy exercises to develop flair with your clients, based on individual need.

TIP 20 – INDIRECT THERAPY

Therapy is usually classified as either direct or indirect, with the former describing specific voice exercises and the latter encompassing vocal hygiene. Healthy voice care is the foundation on which to build effective voice use and when clients leave their initial voice appointment they should be thinking about a new or renewed commitment to optimal voice care.

Across published and locally produced information on voice care, you will see that it usually *encourages* hydration, steam inhalations, or nebulisers, and rest when the voice is tired, and *discourages* throat clearing, smoking, dry atmospheres, and whispering. If your SLT department does not have their own version of a voice care leaflet Martin (2021) provides a good summary of voice care recommendations, as does the Royal College of Speech and Language Therapists and the British Voice Association. The weblinks for the RCSLT's and BVA's factsheets are in the reference list.

Hydration

Hydrating the whole body, or systemic hydration, maintains healthy mucosal tissue and can be achieved by drinking 1 millilitre of water for every calorie burned each day, and for healthy active adults this equates with around 2 litres each day, with more during exercise. Surface, or superficial, hydration of the vocal folds can be achieved through steam inhalations and 0.9% saline nebulisations, complemented by also avoiding drying environments (Alves et al., 2019). With dehydration of mucosal tissue, voices become hoarse and less flexible with compromised pitch and loudness control. In the immediate term, this may mean poorer attempts on the perceptual aspects of your assessment and in the longer term could lead to worsening symptoms and the development of pathologies such as vocal fold nodules.

Historically, caffeinated drinks have been discouraged for their diuretic, or drying, effect, but two systematic reviews have not found strong evidence to suggest it should be avoided (Alves et al., 2019; Georgalas et al., in press). Indeed, where two mugs of strong coffee have a drying effect for one client, they have no impact for another speaker. Caffeine, like the intake of spicy foods and alcohol, needs to be taken in context of the whole picture. If a client is drinking only two cups of coffee, smoking several cigarettes a day, has regular reflux from eating spicy foods, and is complaining of hoarseness, we are likely to recommend increased water intake, reduction in smoking, and consideration of dietary changes. These changes should not only improve their voice but also have a positive impact on their wider health. The mantra of "everything in moderation" is appropriate here (apart from smoking which is never good for you).

When encouraging clients to increase their water intake, do be realistic in your expectations as they are unlikely to progress from drinking three small glasses with their meals one day to two litres the next. Gradually increasing this will feel less daunting and be more likely to bring about success. Free mobile phone apps to log fluid intake may be a helpful reminder for clients who drink little during the day. An increased fluid intake will lead to more frequent trips to the bathroom while the body adjusts, and clients with altered bladder function due to a specific medical condition, age, or childbirth may be reluctant to drink more in places where bathroom facilities are not readily available. You should also be careful if clients are taking on diuretics, commonly described as "water tablets", as they may have been advised to limit their fluid intake for medical reasons. That advice takes precedence over the need to drink more water for the voice as steam inhalations or 0.9% saline nebulisers can be used as a hydrating alternative (Vermeulen et al., 2021).

Mouth breathing also contributes to surface dehydration in the vocal tract and this is particularly relevant for clients who breathe through their mouth at night. Clients don't always know how they breathe when sleeping but the tell-tale sign of at least some nocturnal mouth breathing is snoring. ENT assessment will identify any obstructive reason for nasal breathing such as deviation of the septum or a history of allergies but mouth breathing is to be discouraged where possible.

Avoid throat clearing

Occasional throat clearing is a natural behaviour to clear excessive secretions but habitual throat clearing is damaging to the vocal folds. With a protective epithelial layer, the vocal folds are designed to vibrate gently so slamming them together with harsh throat clearing runs counter to this. Assuming your client has attended for laryngeal assessment, you should know whether there are any excessive secretions around the larynx, remembering that what was visible may be influenced by hydration levels at the time of assessment. Where there isn't a pathology or excessive secretions causing the throat clearing, you should explain to your client that the throat clearing has become habitual, that's not to say that they don't experience a sensation of needing to clear their throat but the more a client clears their throat, the more they're likely to want to clear their throat, and it becomes a vicious circle as in Figure 7.

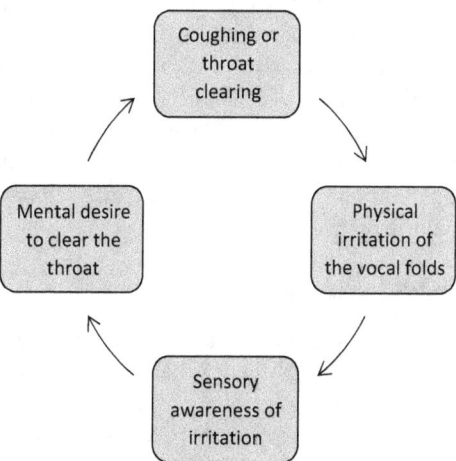

Figure 7 The cycle of throat clearing and irritation

Throat clearing can be relieved by a combination of:

- taking sips of water every time there is an urge to clear their throat. This reduces the feeling of dryness contributing to vocal fold irritation, increases systemic hydration, and brings the vocal folds together more gently when swallowing. Any secretions in the throat will also be cleared through the act of swallowing
- steam inhalations as in self-development activity 4 or 0.9% saline nebulisers
- determination! Once clients are aware of their throat clearing, willpower is needed to resist the temptation to clear the throat and although 30 days is often touted as the time it takes to instil new habits, I've found that habitual throat clearing can be reversed in as little as a week or so with focus

Avoid whispering

In response to emerging voice difficulties some clients start whispering. Seen as a short-term means of voice protection, whispering unfortunately constricts the breath through a narrow channel (compare this to mouthing silently where the air flows freely through the vocal tract) and can lead to a long-term maladaptive habit as with throat clearing. Instead of whispering, voice use should be decreased to a minimum and a confidential voice – a voice as if you're telling someone a secret next to you – should be used instead. It has phonation but is quiet and gentle on the vocal tract.

Wider vocal tract care

Any clients using steroid medication for asthma should be advised to use a spacer with their inhaler, and rinse their mouth with water after use to reduce the drying effects and risk of oropharyngeal candidiasis (thrush). Clients should not swallow the water after rinsing their mouth. I've met many clients who have never been advised by a medical practitioner to rinse after inhaler use so do check this is being done.

Other good voice care practices are picked up later with voice conservation in Tip 29 and smoking cessation in Tips 30 and 48.

TIP 21 – NURTURING A HEALTHY MIND–BODY CONNECTION

We have already acknowledged that we cannot separate the mind–body connection (Tip 14) as swirling thoughts interrupt healthy voice decisions (van Leer, 2021) and contribute to creeping bodily tension, particularly that within the upper body, head, neck, and shoulders. Although observation of physical symptoms alone can't tell us which are related to underlying stress (Behlau et al., in press), we do know that what is contained in the body and mind at large can be reflected in the voice, and unfortunately tension also radiates. Try this experiment: clench your fist and feel the tension not only in your hand but in your forearm, and possibly in your upper arm if you are engaging the rest of your body. Just as tension radiated from your fist up your arm, gross tension in the upper body and around the head and neck can radiate towards the vocal tract and the intrinsic muscles of the voice.

Tip 25 gives an overview of semi-occluded vocal tract exercises which are used to counteract tightness in the vocal tract, and Tips 27 and 28 consider specific diagnoses relating to excessive vocal tension, but here we'll think about the broader management of mind and body tension.

Managing mind tension

Tip 22 explores mindfulness meditation as a means of developing client awareness and it's also a means of managing stress through increased tolerance of "what is" instead of becoming overwhelmed by discomfort. There are several mobile phone apps offering guided meditations and free meditation downloads ranging from three minute breathing spaces to forty-five minute body scans are available at www.freemindfulness.org. Medina and Mead (2021) also include several helpful resources in their paper. Although mindfulness was brought into healthcare to address clinical issues such as chronic pain or addiction, there is good evidence that even low-intensity meditative practice is helpful in improving cognition and perception, emotional regulation, social behaviours, interpersonal processes, and modification of health behaviour (Heppner & Shirk, 2018) so we should all be meditating!

Developing a routine in mindfulness is not always easy – it is, of course, a behavioural change in itself – but with meditations as short as three minutes, these should be accessible to everyone. It is the length of time we might mindlessly (the opposite of being mindful) scroll through social media or the time we wait for the kettle to boil for a hot drink so really we have no excuse. We might exclaim "but I'm so busy I have no time!" and yet it is these moments which reinforce the value of stress management. The more we claim we have no space for meditation, the more likely we are to need it and the more crucial it is to make that space.

Tip 47 considers the professionals involved in supporting mental well-being and if clients are finding it difficult to manage their stress it may be prudent for you to consider onward referral to an appropriate service.

Managing body tension

Easing the troubles of our mind may also extend to benefits for our body – when we feel under less pressure with greater emotion regulation, our bodies carry less tension which, in turn, reduces pressure within the vocal tract. I recall a primary school teacher who booked a monthly massage to uphold good self-care and although we may not be able to afford such a regular luxury, all forms of self-care are important for our wider well-being as well as the voice. To address bodily tension directly, we and our clients can reduce upper body tension with neck stretches such as those in the warm-up guide produced by the British Association of Performing Arts Medicine (Tip 43) and therapists trained in manual therapy for the voice will be able to contribute to tension relief through hands-on practice.

TIP 22 – AWARENESS, AWARENESS, AWARENESS!

Your assessment may have highlighted factors influencing your client's voice which they hadn't noticed before, or hadn't understood as having a link to dysphonia, but developing client awareness can kickstart improved vocal health and vocal growth (Medina & Mead, 2021). Heightened awareness has also been recognised by clients as being important (van Leer & Connor, 2010). For any of us to change we need to be aware of what could be done differently as it's difficult to make any change if we are in pre-contemplation stage, oblivious to our harmful voice behaviours (Tip 4). Clients may need to be aware of their fluid intake, their vocal tract tension, subtle changes in voice quality – the list goes on. Developing awareness can be facilitated in several different ways which are outlined here.

Education

We have a responsibility to highlight negative influences on our clients' voices and guide them towards healthier behaviours. Understanding normal voice function reinforces the importance of good vocal health, and even if you've already explained this in an early therapy session, a later reminder may be helpful, so have a layperson's explanation of the voice at your fingertips (or lips!).

SLT questioning

Questions which prompt clients to discover and describe vocal tract sensations can nurture a more intimate relationship with the voice which subsequently feeds in to the transfer of skills across different situations (Iwarsson, 2015). Our feedback is limited to the clinic room but clients have permanent access to their own sensations so internal awareness is important.

Voice diaries

We don't pay attention to much of our daily life, automatically completing routine activities such as brushing our teeth, but diaries can highlight the extent to which we practice a particular behaviour, compared with how much we *think* we practise it. Mobile phone apps monitor our screen time, food diaries expose what we're really eating, and voice diaries can reinforce just how much vocal exercise we have across individual days or whole weeks. Whether recording your patterns of voice use and care in self-development activity 4 revealed new insights into your voice habits or confirmed what you already knew, it brought awareness to that moment. Depending on your client's needs you can use voice diaries to capture a variety of experiences including: severity of perceived dysphonia; amount of voice use; severity of physical sensations associated with voice change; location of physical sensations; and mood. You could create a personalised diary or use a voice review checklist such as that in Martin (2021).

Negative practice to compare old and new voice

You learnt in Tip 9 that negative practice can support clients to connect with the target voice quality (Iwarsson, 2015) and it is worthwhile placing a reminder here that contrasting voice qualities can consolidate growing awareness and development of the voice.

Meditation

The previous tip introduced meditation as a strategy to manage stress but another prime aim of meditative practice is to develop an openhearted, moment-to-moment, non-judgemental awareness which, as well as generating a relaxed feeling (Medina & Mead, 2021), brings greater attention to the body and mind as "a place we mostly ignore" (Kabat-Zinn, 2005, p. 10). Medina and Mead suggest that mindfulness can aid the development of kinaesthetic, visual, and auditory awareness in voicework and I agree from my experience of using this with clients. I remember one client who attended complaining of toothache but during a short meditative breathing space became aware of a knot in their stomach which reflected their ongoing stress. Without tuning into this feeling, the physical impact of stress may have gone unnoticed and, as a result, unaddressed. At the time of writing, there is not an evidence base for mindfulness in voice therapy specifically but we can draw on the effectiveness from other healthcare disciplines to understand its relevance. The meditation resources highlighted in Tip 21 for stress management are also applicable here including the free online meditations and Medina and Mead's (2021) suggestions.

> **SELF-DEVELOPMENT ACTIVITY 17 – EXPLORING MINDFULNESS YOURSELF**
>
> Use this link to access free downloadable breathing spaces www.freemindfulness.org and then reflect:
>
> - What influenced your choice of breathing space? Length? Purpose? Speaker's voice?
> - What was your experience?
>
> Knowing that mindfulness meditation can be helpful for us all, whether we have voice problems or not, can you try these for a week so you are informed about the possible experience when recommending meditation to your clients?
>
> Note that as there's an emphasis on non-judging in mindfulness there are no right or wrong experiences here. Given that the meditations focus on in-the-moment experiences, you may find your thoughts around practice change from day-to-day, or even from morning to evening, depending on what's going on for you.

Hindsight

Finally, although we're aiming for clients to develop their awareness in the present moment and work proactively with their voice, the adage that hindsight is a wonderful thing is also relevant. Noticing differences in voice quality or production *after* speaking is still awareness and with practice of paying attention to different signals, this should evolve from retrospective hindsight to in-the-moment awareness and onwards to proactive decision-making when speaking.

TIP 23 – HEAR IT, FEEL IT, LOCATE IT

Evaluation of audible voice features can be achieved by using acoustic software, our ears, and our clients' ears. Our clients additionally have unique access to internal sensations and we should exploit the opportunity to develop their awareness of what, where, and how these inhabit their body. Let's consider how our clients can sense the voice to expand their awareness and nurture their skills in being their own therapist.

Hearing

A negative change in the sound of the voice is a signal to the client that they need to pay attention and modify voice behaviour or vocal health. Conversely, positive changes in voice quality or sensations highlight what should be done more often to maintain and expand effective voice production. Client awareness of audible features can be developed through obvious questions such as "what did you hear in that sound?" or "what did you pick up on, listening to your voice in that conversation?" and then more deeply by encouraging clients to identify discrepancies between different sounds, activities, or elements of conversation. At times, the evaluation will simply be based on the presence or absence of hoarseness or strain, and at others it will be more advanced in considering the extent of forward tone or different resonant qualities.

Feeling

Limiting voice evaluation to audible features risks missing pertinent information so this should be complemented by what the client feels. We can ask clients to notice a particular sensation, to evaluate a sensation, or compare different sensations (Madill et al., 2020). In fact, sometimes paying attention to sensations can be more important than listening out for voice changes – clients with vocal fatigue, for example, may perceptively have a normal voice quality but if fatigue is contributing to increased effort, vocal function is compromised. Additionally, a reliance on audible features is a limiting evaluative measure for difficulties which heal over time. For example, if the conversational voice of a client with vocal fold nodules is rated as $G_2 R_2 B_1 A_1 S_1$ at the start of an appointment, they may leave the session with the same roughness and breathiness rating, as nodules do not resolve within 45 minutes. Paying gentle attention to muscular sensations and noticing a reduction in strain, however, would be more useful evidence of change. A further example would be pre-operative voice therapy for a client with laryngeal papillomas. As improved laryngeal appearance is reliant on surgery, the voice will not return to normal within a single therapy session, but if we also consider how therapy addresses secondary muscle tension dysphonia, there could be detectable positive changes in vocal tract sensation before their operation.

As clients normalise altered voice qualities or sensations, it becomes more difficult to detect changes from day to day, both when the voice sounds a little easier and when it is a little more difficult. The ability to notice different sensations is important though to avoid altered qualities or sensations becoming embedded, or further embedded, as the more familiar way of speaking.

Locating

Beyond feeling the general presence of a sensation in the vocal system, the ability to identify where this is located adds another, sophisticated layer of attention to guide therapy. Locating a sensation is relevant in noticing both negative sensations to reduce, such as jaw tension, and positive reflections of the voice to maintain. Feeling and locating are not solely focused on what is not working well. As negative sensations ease, a client may comment that they feel nothing at all but rather than feeling *nothing*, they're expressing awareness of greater space, for example, which is a sensation in itself.

TIP 24 – JUST BREATHE...

The breath is consistently referenced in theoretical texts, therapy resources, and clinical voice frameworks for good reason – it powers vocal fold vibration and the voice is impacted by some respiratory conditions. The breath is second only to a tension-free body in Shewell's (2009) framework and as the fundamental energy source, breathwork may seem a logical starting point for therapy. For some clients it may be, but do not be lured into thinking this is the starting point for all clients as it is not warranted if there is no maladaptive breathing style (Iwarsson, 2015). When planning therapy we need to ask ourselves if issues which seem to be breath-related are really a contributing factor or if the difficulties are related to other elements in the vocal system. Phonation is shaped by whatever it meets during exhalation so if the breath "meets" a palsied vocal fold, increased breath flows through the wider glottic gap and contributes to a breathier quality. If it "meets" tensely adducted false cords, it will contribute to the strained quality of ventricular phonation, or if it "meets" vocal fold nodules, its passage will be interrupted by the pathology and contribute to characteristic roughness.

Tip 33 considers the breath in relation to upper airway disorders but here we will consider the following aspects of breath work:

- improved coordination of the breath and phonation
- improved breath placing
- improved phrasing
- greater relaxation
- developing an anchoring point in meditation

Improved coordination of the breath and phonation

Some clients ask whether they should breathe through their mouth or nose and there is a two-fold response to account for breathing at rest and breathing during speaking. Alongside the drying effect from mouth breathing (Tip 14) it also increases respiratory exertion which can lead to general shortness of breath, poorer lung function, and feelings of stress. By contrast, breathing through the nose moistens, warms, and filters the air and should therefore be encouraged at rest.

When speaking it is more time-efficient to take top-up breaths through the mouth as we don't have time in our short pauses for slower nasal inhalations. As clients work to increase the frequency of oral inhalations during conversations, there can be a temptation to say a few words, stop for breath, and only once this is replenished do they restart the utterance. In reality, our articulators anticipate the oral placement required for the next clause and start moving while the breath is being inhaled for a more seamless process. Try it for yourself!

Improved breath placing

A high intercostal or clavicular breathing style contributes to upper body tension through over-recruitment of our secondary respiratory muscles, the sternocleidomastoids, and for singers and actors can lead to performance anxiety. Conversely, a breath located lower in the body, and further away from the phonatory source, reduces the likelihood that tension inhibits the neck and laryngeal muscles (Iwarsson, 2015). Clients can adapt their breathing patterns by consciously placing their breath lower and then allowing their body to settle in to this new cycle of inhalation and exhalation. During specific practice, lying on a bed or the floor with a box of tissues on their stomach can be useful feedback to identify where the breath should be as they take time to retrain a maladaptive breathing pattern.

Improved phrasing

As a general rule, running out of breath during conversations leads to laryngeal strain to maintain phonation and therefore should be avoided. Your initial voice evaluation should note any differences in breath between single sounds, a reading passage and conversational speech, and you may observe bigger breath groups – that is, a greater number of words said per breath – in spontaneous conversation than during a reading task where punctuation highlights the places to pause and inhale. Unfortunately bigger breath groups in a fast rate of speech reduce the frequency of inhalations, shorten the inhalation taken, and lead to glottal compression and strain (Kuhlmann & Iwarsson, in press) so this is not a habit to encourage.

Where clients don't intuitively pause we can use phrases of increasing length to show where breaths could be taken to replenish airflow and such practice also indirectly slows the rate of speech. The suggested phrases below, with the number of syllables at the end of each statement, are in Appendix 2 for you to use with any client. You can also create your own for variety of home practice and you will see in Tips 41 and 42 how this exercise can be personalised for vocal athletes.

There isn't a magic, fully evidence-based number of syllables to allocate to each breath as this will depend on the utterance, conversational context, and the client's individual respiratory function, but I often find that healthy adults with no significant respiratory conditions should be thinking about taking a breath after about ten to thirteen syllables in connected speech. Going by this principle, we should be able to reach the third sentence below with one breath but should be considering a second breath in the fourth sentence which conveniently contains two clauses, one for each breath.

> *I went for a walk* (5)
> *I went for a walk today* (7)
> *I went for a walk today across the fields* (11)
> *I went for a walk today across the fields and it was sunny* (16)
> *I went for a walk today across the fields and it was sunny and hot* (18)
> *I went for a walk today across the fields and it was sunny and hot with a good view* (22)

> *I went for a walk today across the fields and it was sunny and hot with a good view of the countryside* (27)
>
> *I went for a walk today across the fields and it was sunny and hot with a good view of the countryside so I rested on a rock* (34)
>
> *I went for a walk today across the fields and it was sunny and hot with a good view of the countryside so I rested on a rock and drank some water* (39)
>
> *I went for a walk today across the fields and it was sunny and hot with a good view of the countryside so I rested on a rock and drank some cool and refreshing water* (44)

Relaxation

Given calm environmental conditions, guided breathing exercises can be relaxing with gentle, rhythmic inhalations and exhalations settling the mind and allowing body tension to dissipate. Positive imagery can be used to guide clients into a space which feels free of pressure and such exercises can be used in the clinic or by clients independently as part of a regular self-care routine.

Developing an anchoring point in meditation

Although relaxation is not a key aim of meditation, there can be an overlapping relaxing effect, and several clients have commented that meditating just before going to bed seems to generate a better night's sleep. Rather than a focus of relaxation, however, meditation uses the breath as an anchoring point because the breath is the one thing that is always with us. Our thoughts evolve from the beginning to the end of a day, from the beginning of a therapy session to when we say goodbye or from the beginning of a meditative space to the time when we open our eyes, but the breath is always there and as such becomes a consistent place to return to. When our mind wanders during meditative practice, guiding our attention gently, but firmly, back to the breath can re-ground us and develop our skills in focusing. Tip 22 addresses meditation in more depth as a means of developing awareness and there are links to meditations you can try yourself.

TIP 25 – SEMI-OCCLUDED VOCAL TRACT THERAPY

Although I explained in the Introduction that I did not intend to provide every possible therapy exercise, semi-occluded vocal tract (SOVT) exercises deserve inclusion for their growing evidence base and benefit in resetting the voice for speakers and singers, with and without dysphonia (e.g. Cardoso et al., 2020; Kaneko et al., 2020, Zenari et al., in press). In short, SOVT exercises improve vocal economy, efficiency, and intensity (Mills et al., 2018) so phonation is uninterrupted by tension in the vocal tract. They can be active in which the client uses their own mechanical control, such as vibrating their lips, to develop vocal economy, or passive, in which an external mechanism creates the same effect. Let's take a look at both.

Active SOVT exercises

Yawning

As a vegetative behaviour, yawning acts as a conduit to easier phonation by reducing conscious, potentially distracting, thoughts about voicing – sometimes *not* thinking about voice production is what leads to an improved technique. Shewell (2009) provides a very helpful radiological image of vocal tract expansion during a yawn and, although this book is written for practitioners, I do sometimes grab it mid-session to show the image as emphasis of what we're aiming for. Remember in Tip 9 that it's helpful for clients to understand why they're doing what they're doing, and given they can't see inside their vocal tract as we demonstrate exercises, this is an alternative way of showing the target.

Watching someone else yawn can prompt our own yawn so a demonstration from you may generate a yawn for your client, and even thinking about it can be helpful – I feel a yawn developing as I type this section! That said, it can still be difficult for clients to yawn "to command", though you might find that fatigued clients at the start or end of the day can more easily access this.

When yawning silently or with an audible but voiceless sigh, check that the breath is not constricted before adding phonation – if the breath is constricted, it will be more difficult to add phonation without that being constricted too. My description is that clients are aiming for a leisurely, easy-sounding voice and perhaps one that might be attributed to Winnie-the-Pooh, as a character well-known across the age range. If you can think of an alternative character that works for you, please use it.

Lip trills

These were mentioned in Tip 16 as a quick way of evaluating the stimulability of a client's voice and these can also be used as a specific therapy exercise. Out of curiosity, I've sometimes tried lip trills when I've felt a globus sensation from stress or distress (what a voice geek!) and they're certainly more difficult in these circumstances. Remember that tension radiates (Tip 21) so the laryngeal tightness arising from my discomfort extends the length of the vocal tract, hindering lip trilling. If clients find lip trills challenging, return to Tip 16 for the facilitative strategies.

Humming

Humming is a gentle and easy-to-teach exercise which can be used in post-operative rehabilitation (Tip 36) and as a warm-up exercise (Tip 45) in addition to supporting gentle vocal fold adduction. Proprioceptive feedback through vibrations or tickling in the nose, face, and lips helps clients to locate forward placement of the voice alongside thinking about talking "where you hum and not where you gargle". An /m/ without forward movement and buzz on your lips loses richness and depth, and may sound a little hollow. The negative practice outlined in Tip 9 can highlight differences between easier and more effortful voice production, and facilitate greater vocal control so try self-development activity 18 so you can hear and feel the difference before introducing this to a client.

> **SELF-DEVELOPMENT ACTIVITY 18 – HUMMING**
>
> Try humming yourself.
>
> - Can you feel the buzz, vibration, or tickling on your lips?
> - Can you try negative practice where you don't feel the buzz by holding on to the sound or "tethering it"? Your voice will start to sound like it's only coming from the throat rather than reverberating round the cave of your mouth.

Other SOVT exercises include using voiceless fricatives to establish easy breath flow followed by voiced fricatives to facilitate easy phonation. For the voice newbie, it can be daunting to know which exercise to pick but as well as being influenced by either your mentor or practice educator, give yourself permission to try a range of SOVT strategies – where lip trills click for one client, others will find humming to be more informative so there is no single right answer.

Passive SOVT exercises

Using straws or tubes, with and without water, artificially narrows and extends the length of the vocal tract to create a massaging back pressure which reduces vocal stress (Cardoso et al., 2020). Hard-walled straws may give greater feedback in terms of vibration round the lips but silicone tubes may have a marginally stronger massaging effect on the vocal folds (Tyrmi et al., 2017). For non-elite voice users, there is likely to be little difference in outcome between using a paper straw or metal straw, but buying disposable plastic straws is to be discouraged from an environmental perspective.

As with any therapeutic exercise you need to be able to increase and decrease the level of difficulty to facilitate vocal mastery. This can be achieved through changing the length or diameter of the straw but the most useful combination for any client will be found through experimentation as our individual vocal tract pressures are different, and therefore one size does not fit all. Some specifically designed straws have adaptable diameters and lengths but you can replicate this yourself by using paper straws of different widths and cutting them to different lengths. Placing the tube in water and placing it lower in the water further increases the resistance for development of practice.

Which are more effective – passive or active exercises?

Continued practice of any of these exercises beyond a defined period of therapy can help to maintain optimal function of the voice and be used as part of a warm-up routine (Zenari et al., in press). Passive SOVT practice may have more replicable results as the straw is the constant facilitator of easy phonation, unlike active SOVT exercises where the client needs to control the output but this doesn't mean that active trills are ineffective or should be avoided. Being able to maintain a voluntary lip trill, for example, is evidence of improved vocal control and there is advantage in being able to practise this anywhere and anytime without the need for equipment.

> **SELF-DEVELOPMENT ACTIVITY 19 – SOVT PRACTICE**
>
> Try a week of using SOVT exercises and see what you notice in your voice.
>
> - Are they helpful to reset your voice and prepare it for the day?
> - You can also use this experiment as another opportunity to reflect on your connection with change as in self-development activity 8. Did you feel ready

> for the challenge when reading the suggestion above or did you groan out loud? Remember that whatever thought you had, there's a client somewhere who has had, or will have, that thought too!

TIP 26 – BREAK IT DOWN OR BUILD IT UP?

With any client our long-term aim will be for the transfer of skills across different speaking situations and this is achieved through consistent practice which is neither too easy and generates little benefit, nor too challenging in compounding the existing problem. Practice can be approached from either a bottom-up or top-down perspective.

Working bottom-up

Here practice is organised hierarchically so early tasks focus on the simplest elements of voice and are then extended through gradually increased complexity of task. This "decomposing complex behaviour" (Iwarsson, 2015) can be done through segmentation, fractionation, simplification, and the development of automaticity. They are presented individually here, but in reality can be combined so automatic phrases, for example, could be blended with segmentation as a bridge between words, phrases, and sentence.

Segmentation

Production starts at phoneme level and is extended to CV, VC, CVC, VCV combinations, multisyllabic words, phrases, longer sentences, and finally, conversation. Each time a client progresses to a new level of practice you will remind them of what learning they need to bring through from previous practice.

Fractionation

This approach considers individual elements of speaking so breathing, for example, is addressed separately from phonation. Some clients do benefit from a fractionated approached though Tip 19 highlighted the opportunities to treat multiple subsystems with a single exercise, and Tip 24 encouraged you to think carefully about your rationale for breathing exercises.

Simplification

Here practice is adapted to facilitate easier phonation. Breathing when lying on the floor or using full body movements to reduce tension can maintain easier voicing (Shewell, 2009; Iwarsson 2015) even if the strategies may not immediately seem facilitative – swirling round a room while voicing might seem counter-intuitive but it can loosen the body and reduce any unhelpful focus on the larynx. Try it!

Development of automaticity

In the earlier stages of therapy, client focus on how they can achieve the target behaviour will be high but, in time, they should achieve the same target without excessive cognitive load. Automaticity can be developed through a hierarchy of automatic phrases (such as days of the week or months of the year), repeated phrases in a set form (I see a…, I like a…), listing words (such as names of animals), answering simple questions, and finally semi-spontaneous speech. This temporary increase in cognitive load embeds the new voice production strategies before new skills are habitual with low cognitive load.

Working top-down

In contrast with a bottom-up approach, Conversation Training Therapy (CTT) (Gartner-Schmidt & Gillespie, 2021) uses client-led conversation as the practice stimulus. The rationale is that generalisation can be the most challenging aspect of voice therapy (van Leer & Connor, 2010), but in coming last in a bottom-up sequence of practice tasks, the client is left without an optimally functioning voice for most of their therapy experience. Using motor-learning principles, Garner-Schmidt and Gillespie argue that CTT:

- activates all parts of conversational speech (*whole-practice learning*)
- improves learning through the greater *cognitive effort* required to use new voice skills at conversational level

- exploits the real-life nature of conversational practice and therefore there is *contextual relevance* of practice
- improves learning by acknowledging the variable nature of conversation (*schema theory*)
- ensures practice is relevant, with *salience and specificity* so non-speech exercises, which may not appear to be relevant to conversation for the client, are avoided.

Iwarsson's (2015) "each time – every time" principle applies here in encouraging clients to use their voice learning every time they speak for greater vocal stability. The risk, as Iwarsson acknowledges, is that spontaneous conversation away from the clinic will not be subject to the same level of control as is possible in a therapy room, and I can recall clients who achieved successful voice production within specific practice but struggled to maintain this during the rest of the week. It can certainly be more difficult to integrate new skills in the face of environmental or emotional challenges such as a faster-paced conversation, a rush to answer the phone, or safety issues requiring a rapid response. Although van Leer and Connor (2010) identify cognitive effort as a potential hindrance to therapy, Gartner-Schmidt and Gillespie attempt to capitalise on this in CTT.

So which one do I choose?

Ultimately, neither approach is more right than the other. If we are client-centred and respond to individual needs, and if we remember there is an art and craft to voice therapy, we may need to interweave both top-down and bottom-up components in our practice. For some of my clients the systematic layering of skills in bottom-up thinking extended their learning from one level to another, and the greater phonatory ease they achieved on vowels helped their transfer of skills to word level. Conversely, but as commonly, some of my clients felt practising single words was false and led to unnatural intonation but short, functional phrases and conversation facilitated practice of communication in a context more reflective of real life. Furthermore, I can think of clients who gained confidence from easier vowel phonation but the message then spontaneously clicked that they could try using the same way of speaking in conversation before I'd got to the point of explaining that!

Even when adopting a hierarchical approach to practice, I still encourage clients to at least consider how their learning at a simple level can be applied to conversation, as a means of increasing their awareness (Tip 22). If a client is able to achieve easier or stronger phonation at a CV, CVC, or word level, can they notice what is different when they say "good morning" to their family or enquire after a friend's well-being? The ease with which clients produce voice in the clinic is the same ease I want them to have during the rest of the week and across the different voice contexts.

Regardless of how you approach generalisation of new skills, the ultimate aim is to develop more frequent use of effective voice production. Using the analogy of weighing scales, at the start of therapy a more difficult voice is more present and therefore weighs more heavily, and the easier voice is comparatively lighter as in Figure 8a below.

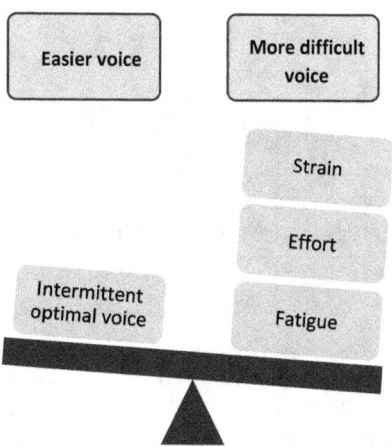

Figure 8a A more difficult voice weighs more heavily before therapy

Through therapy and practice, the easier and difficult voices reach a stage where they are used equally as in Figure 8b.

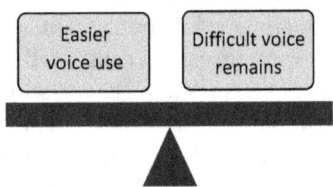

Figure 8b More equally weighted use of effective and less effective voice use

Finally, by the end of therapy you are aiming for the easier voice to be used most of the time as in Figure 8c.

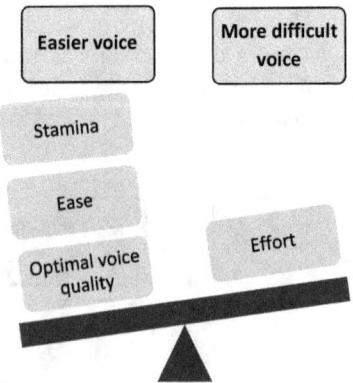

Figure 8c Effective voice outweighs ineffective voice use

REFERENCES

Alves, M., Krüger, E., Pillay, B., van Lierde, K. & van der Linde, J. (2019) The Effect of Hydration on Voice Quality in Adults: A Systematic Review. *Journal of Voice 33* (1) 125.e13–125.e28 https://doi.org/10.1016/j.jvoice.2017.10.001

Behlau, M., Madazio, G., Pacheco, C., Vaiano, T., Badaró, F. & Barbara, M. (in press) Coaching Strategies for Behavioural Voice Therapy and Training. *Journal of Voice* https://doi.org/10.1016/j.jvoice.2020.12.039

Cardoso, N. S, V., Lucena, J. A., Gomes, A de O. C (2020) Immediate Effect of a Resonance Tube on the Vocal Range Profile of Choristers. *Journal of Voice 43* (5) 667–674 https://doi.org/10.1016/j.jvoice.2019.01.006

Ebersole, B., Soni, R. S., Moran, K., Lango, M., Devarajan, K. & Jamal, N. (2017) The Influence of Occupation on Self-perceived Vocal Problems in Patients With Voice Complaints. *Journal of Voice 32* (6) 673–680 https://doi.org/10.1016/j.jvoice.2017.08.028

Gartner-Schmidt, J. & Gillespie, A. I. (2021) Conversation Training Therapy: Let's Talk It Through. *Seminars in Speech and Language 42* (1) 32–40 10.1055/s-0040-1722751

Georgalas, V. L., Kalantzi, N., Harpur, I. & Kenny, C. (in press) The Effects of Caffeine on Voice: A Systematic Review. *Journal of Voice* https://doi.org/10.1016/j.jvoice.2021.02.025

Heppner, W. L. & Shirk, S. D. (2018) Mindful Moments: A Review of Brief, Low-Intensity Mindfulness Meditation and Induced Mindful States. *Social and Personality Psychology Compass 12* (12) e12424 https://doi.org/10.1111/spc3.12424

Iwarsson, J. (2015) Facilitating Behavioral Learning and Habit Change in Voice Therapy –Theoretic Premises and Practical Strategies. *Logopedics Phoniatrics Vocology 40* (4) 179–186 https://doi.org/10.3109/14015439.2014.936498

Kabat-Zinn, J. (2005) *Coming To Our Senses. Healing Ourselves and the World Through Mindfulness*. London: Piatkus

Kaneko, M., Sugiyama, Y., Mukudai, S. & Hirano, S. (2020) Effect of Voice Therapy Using Semioccluded |Vocal Tract Exercises in Singers and Nonsingers with Dysphonia. *Journal of Voice 34* (6) 963.e1–963.e9 https://doi.org/10.1016/j.j.voice.2019.06.014

Kuhlmann, L. L. & Iwarsson, J. (in press) Effects of Speaking Rate on Breathing and Voice Behavior. *Journal of Voice* https://doi.org/10.1016/j.jvoice.2021.09.005

Madill, C., Chacom, A., Kirby, E., Novakovic, D. & Nguyenm D. D. (2021) Active Ingredients of Voice Therapy for Muscle Tension Voice Disorders: A Retrospective Data Audit. *Journal of Clinical Medicine 10* (18) 4135 https://doi.org/10.3390/jcm10184135

Madill, C., McIlwaine, A., Russell, R., Hodges, N. J. & McCabe, P. (2020) Classifying and Identifying Motor Learning Behaviors in Voice-Therapy Clinician-Client Interactions: A Proposed Motor Learning Classification Framework. *Journal of Voice 34* (5) 806.e19–806.e31 https://doi.org/10.1016/j,jvoice.2019.03.014

Martin, S. (2021) *Working With Voice Disorders. Theory and Practice.* (3rd Ed.) Abingdon: Routledge

Medina, A. M. & Mead, J. S. (2021) An Exploration of Mindfulness in Speech-Language Pathology. *Communication Disorders Quarterly 42* (4) 257–265 https://doi.org/10.1177/1525740120942141

Mills, R. D., Rivedal, S., DeMorett, C., Maples, G. & Jiang, J. J. (2018) Effects of Straw Phonation Through Tubes of Varied Lengths on Sustained Vowels in Normal-Voiced Participants. *Journal of Voice 32* (3) 386.e21–386.e29 https://doi.org/10.1016/j.jvoice.2017.05.015

Shewell, C. (2009) *Voice Work. Art and Science in Changing Voices.* Chichester: Wiley-Blackwell

Tyrmi, J., Radolf, V., Horáček, J. & Laukkanen, A-M. (2017) Resonance Tube or Lax Vox? *Journal of Voice 31* (4) 430–437 https://doi.org/10.1016/j.jvoice.2016.10.024

van Leer, E. (2021) Enhancing Adherence to Voice Therapy via Social Cognitive Strategies. *Seminars in Speech and Language 42* (1) 19–31 https://doi.org/10.1055/s-0040-1722755

van Leer, E. & Connor, N. P. (2010) Patient Perceptions of Voice Therapy Adherence. *Journal of Voice 24* (4) 458–469 https://doi.org/10.1016/j.jvoice.2008.12.009.

Vermeulen, R., van der Linde, J., Abdoola, S., van Lierde, K. & Graham, M. A. (2021) The Effect of Superficial Hydration, With or Without Systemic Hydration, on Voice Quality in Future Female Professional Singers. *Journal of Voice* 35 (5) 728–738 https://doi.org.10.1016/j.jvoice.2020.01.008

Zenari, M. S., dos Reis Cota, A. de Albuquerque Rodrigues, D. & Nemr, K. (in press) Do Professionals Who Use the Voice in a Journalistic Context Benefit from Humming as a Semi-occluded Vocal Tract Exercise? *Journal of Voice* https://doi.org/10.1016/j.jvoice.2021.03.011

ADDITIONAL LEARNING RESOURCES

Royal College of Speech and Language Therapists' voice care factsheet www.rcslt.org/wp-content/uploads/2020/07/rcslt-voice-care-factsheet.pdf

British Voice Association's voice care factsheet www.britishvoiceassociation.org.uk/voicecare_take-care-of-your-voice.htm

Free Mindfulness www.freemindfulness.org/download

Chapter 6

WORKING WITH SPECIFIC DIAGNOSES

In this chapter you will learn about the key aspects of therapy in relation to 13 different voice diagnoses. We will consider those without pathology (functional voice disorder and psychogenic voice disorder), diagnoses with physiological changes for which voice therapy is the first line of defence (vocal fold nodules, Reinke's oedema, granulomas, vocal fold palsies, upper airway disorders, and presbyphonia) and diagnoses which usually require surgical intervention (spasmodic dysphonia, laryngeal papillomas, polyps, and cysts). Alongside the usual focus of therapy, each diagnosis is introduced with its typical vocal qualities and common causes. Becoming familiar with the characteristic voice qualities of each diagnosis makes it easier to identify unexpected presentations, formulate a working hypothesis and plan therapy.

TIP 27 – FUNCTIONAL VOICE DISORDER

> *Typical voice quality*: rough, strained, and weak with reduced stamina. There may also be a globus sensation.
>
> *Common causes*: poor habitual voice production or maladaptive response to hoarseness arising from another condition. There may also be reported emotional stress but this is not the main influencing factor on the voice.
>
> *Treatment*: direct and indirect voice therapy with a focus on reducing vocal tract tension. Medical intervention may be required if there are co-existing or contributing medical conditions such as asthma or reflux.

Tip 17 introduced the possibility of new terminology around functional voice disorder (Hacki et al., 2022) but as that has yet to change I shall use the current terms here.

Primary muscle tension dysphonia

Functional voice disorder (FVD) is sub-divided into primary muscle tension dysphonia (MTD), caused by excessive circumlaryngeal tension without any organic change to the vocal folds, and secondary MTD which occurs in response to organic or neurological changes (Madill et al., 2021). In simple terms, this means there are no "lumps or bumps" to see on ENT examination with primary MTD, though repeated throat clearing or coughing may lead to a general picture of laryngeal irritation. Significant MTD may include inward movement of the false cords which can obstruct the view of the true vocal folds. Where there is no visible pathology on flexible nasendoscopy or videostroboscopy, diagnosis is made based on clinical evaluation of the voice and client data.

In addition to voice changes there may be hyperextension of the head and neck, shortened and compressed respiration, a high laryngeal position and tension within the face (Dehqan &

Scherer, 2019). Although the larynx benefits from movement up and down the vertical plane to retain flexibility, remaining in an elevated position for long periods is tiring and requires effort. Vocal tract discomfort may extend to a globus sensation as if something is stuck in the throat. A phonatory gap (a posterior gap between the true vocal folds) is often linked with weakness but can also be the result of tension.

The development of primary MTD is usually gradual, originating from anticipation of difficulty or a speaker's feeling that they have to give more of the voice to be heard. In adding more effort to sustain the voice, a trajectory of increasing tension begins as additional effort ultimately makes the voice feel weaker and prompts further effort or strain. Like throat clearing, it becomes a cumulative problem and can ultimately lead to aphonia. Figure 9 represents this cumulative effect.

There are no units attached to the time axis as the principle of ever-increasing tension can be applied to a variety of situations – the steps could reflect each hour of a teacher's working day or each day of a salesperson's working week. There is also no defined unit of tension but this is not required for a pictorial representation of tension development for use with clients. These two client examples demonstrate how primary MTD may develop in reality.

Example 1 – a retired computer engineer threw themselves into Rotary and Church commitments a year ago to fill the gap of employment and now has long periods of speaking at once-weekly meetings. Unused to long periods of speaking, they use effortful voice production in these situations to see themselves through and then attempt to recover with voice rest during the rest of the day. This all leads to vocal strain and a lower mood from experiencing difficulty in the few speaking situations they're involved in.

Example 2 – a librarian living with their dog does not have high vocal demands at work but had a winter cold and sore throat which was relieved by the pain relief in regular throat lozenges. Reliance on the lozenges masked their vocal vulnerability and they persisted with effortful use

WORKING WITH SPECIFIC DIAGNOSES 125

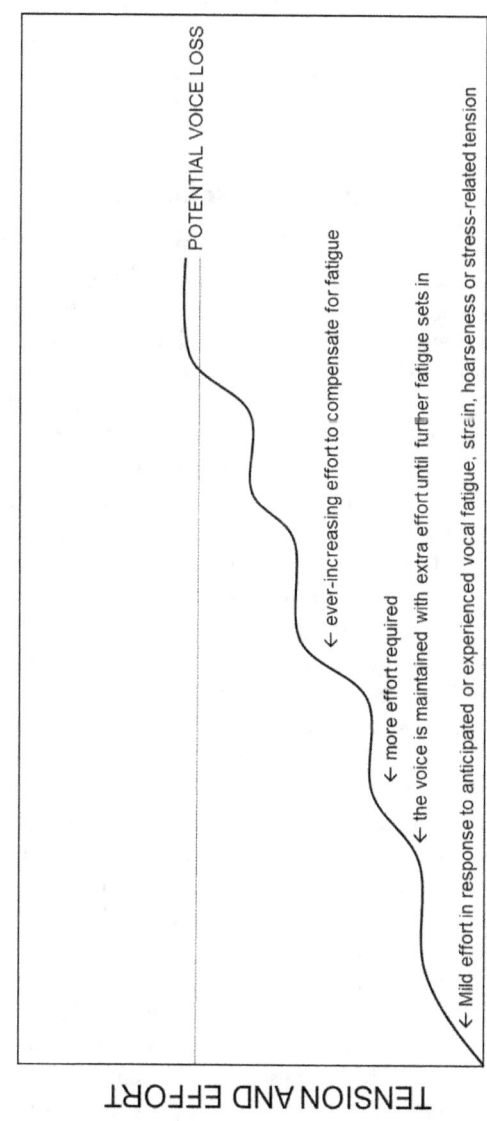

Figure 9 The cumulative effect of tension with the voice

of the voice in damp weather to call the dog. The laryngeal tension was exacerbated by upper body tension from a hunched, protective posture from being cold during the walk and from feeling unwell, and poor sitting posture from home working compounded the problem.

Secondary muscle tension dysphonia

Secondary MTD follows a similar pattern of cumulative difficulty but occurs in response to existing difficulties which could relate to a gradual process such as slowly recurring papillomas, or an isolated event such as a voice break during a performance.

Taking this out of SLT for a moment to provide an example, imagine you've sprained your ankle but your work, commute, or a hobby relies on movement. Although the sore ankle doesn't prevent you from walking completely, it does make it harder and more uncomfortable so you try to find an alternative way of moving. This might include a greater reliance on your non-injured side or walking more gingerly on the injured side, but whatever you do, your compensatory way of moving starts to become a problem in itself. The more you walk in this new way, the more you become accustomed to it. Meanwhile, your sprain is healing nicely and soon there are no ill-effects from it, other than your new, imbalanced way of walking and a growing risk of low mood and depression from a new issue.

Bringing this back to SLT, when clients experience difficulty with their voice they may consciously or unconsciously adopt new ways of speaking but as the strategy is maladaptive, it either compounds the issue directly related to the pathology or generates a new voice problem. In the examples at the start of this section, this might mean that the client with papillomas finds it difficult to regain a normal voice quality post-surgery as they now automatically produce voice with effort, or the worry around future voice breaks leads to a cautious approach to singing which negatively impacts both the client's technique and their experience of performing, as neatly captured in the fear-avoidance model (Leeuw et al., 2007).

In real terms, this might mean:

Example 3 – a student of French was diagnosed with vocal fold nodules shortly before their exams which included oral assessment of their language proficiency. Worried about not being able to complete their exams, and not yet attending SLT, they chose to rest their voice and started whispering instead. Although the infection resolved and they felt better in themselves, they struggled to regain their voice once the whispering-related tension became embedded as their new voice quality.

Example 4 – a customer care assistant with Reinke's oedema is finding it difficult to call to colleagues across the shop floor. In a bid to maintain a functioning voice they add strain to an already deep-sounding voice from the vocal fold oedema at work.

Indirect therapy

Here and with all other diagnoses, you will use case history information to guide your recommendations regarding vocal care. As mentioned in Tip 20, optimal vocal health is required as a solid foundation for direct therapy exercises.

Direct therapy

The key aim of therapy is to reduce circumlaryngeal tension and early MTD intervention is recommended to prevent maladaptive vocal behaviours becoming ingrained (Madill et al., 2021). Ranking a tension-free body and tension-free vocal tract highly in Shewell's (2009) framework (1st and 3rd places, respectively) reflects the importance of addressing tightness, and particularly addressing gross bodily tension before addressing tension in the smaller muscles of the larynx. It will be difficult to reduce laryngeal tension if a client's shoulders are up round their ears but once bodily tension is low deconstriction exercises, which may include SOVT activities (Tip 25), will be central to your plan. Practice of exercises to alleviate tension will be enhanced if they are accompanied by high-quality feedback (Tip 10) and increased client awareness of their own patterns of tension (Tip 22) so the line in Figure 9 does not continue in an upward trajectory.

Manual circumlaryngeal therapy involves direct, gentle movement and massage of the areas around the larynx to reduce excessive tension. It requires training in order to do this safely but positive effects have been seen in improving vocal fold vibration and a reduction in tension and hoarseness (Dehqan & Scherer, 2019; Aghadoost et al., 2020).

Muscle Tension Dysphagia

Any case history should routinely enquire about swallowing difficulties and this is particularly relevant in MTD in case this is accompanied by muscle tension dysphagia (MTDg). Complaints of eating, drinking, and swallowing difficulties should always be addressed through appropriate assessment to rule out neurological or structural aetiologies. Like its sister voice diagnosis, there may be little to see on objective assessment such as videofluoroscopy, but there may be visible muscle tension on laryngoscopy and therapy focuses on reducing this tension. From clinical experience and early research (Kang et al., 2021) laryngeal deconstriction exercises can be as effective for MTDg as they are for MTD, and circumlaryngeal manual therapy may also be appropriate for clinicians trained in this approach.

TIP 28 – PSYCHOGENIC VOICE DISORDER

> *Typical voice quality*: rough, strained, weak, and there may be an unnaturally high pitch. Some clients will be aphonic in conversation but phonation can be elicited via coughing, laughing, or crying. There may be excessive body tension.
>
> *Common causes*: although there may be poor habitual voice production or vocal care, emotional stress is the main contributing factor.
>
> *Treatment*: indirect therapy to improve voice care generally and therapy to reduce vocal tract tension, but voice therapy alone is unlikely to resolve the problem. Liaison with other health professionals with respect to the client's mental well-being is probable.

The picture on endoscopic evaluation of the larynx is similar in primary muscle tension dysphonia (Tip 27) and psychogenic voice disorder (PVD) in that there is an absence of pathology accompanied by any or all of the following symptoms: poor vocal fold adduction; false cord adduction (ventricular phonation); a globus sensation (a feeling of something stuck in the throat); and excessive muscle tension. Differential diagnosis emerges from the client's report of stressors, a defined onset, and the ability to achieve phonation through non-communicative voicing which all point to PVD. Explaining that the client's difficulties are considered to be psychogenic in origin requires sensitivity and Baker et al. (2021) provide helpful statements as to how to do this, including explanations around the function of the larynx in self-protection and how that can hinder its role in phonation.

Indirect therapy

As with all clients, advice regarding vocal care should be provided where warranted – for example, a client may find solace from stress in smoking or alcohol but you should still advise against this, with recognition that a reduction of the use of these substances may be more difficult at times of heightened stress.

Direct therapy

Given that clients with PVD may be able to phonate through non-communicative situations, therapy uses this as a lead-in to developing more consistent phonation. Using vegetative phonation as a "back door" route can reduce the pressure to achieve successful voicing for conversation, and some clients may be able to achieve normal voice within the first session. Others will need several sessions supported by counselling.

So how is voicing facilitated? A gentle, voiced cough can be developed to include a voiced vowel and then extended into a voiced sigh without reliance on the stimulus cough. Alternatively, a chewing action with the jaw can be enhanced through the addition of an "appreciative mm", as if eating something tasty and, if successful, this can later include pitch variation. Once phonation is established at a basic level, it can be developed using the different routes in Tip 26.

In addition to their helpful suggestions for explaining PVD to a client, Baker et al. (2021) provide further suggestions of how to elicit voice and address the psychological aspects. I would highly recommend you read this article if working with a client with psychogenic dysphonia.

Looking after the client's well-being

In Tip 7 we considered how to support tender conversations and respond when clients share personal information. Although many clients acknowledge life stressors, for clients with PVD these stressors are more significant and/or have a magnified impact. You may hear details of highly sensitive situations including financial worries, the burden and guilt around caring for a loved one, an ongoing divorce, workplace bullying, or abusive relationships and all should be treated with respect and sensitivity, remembering that some clients will be interested in exploring the psychosocial aspects of their voice difficulties and others will not (Baker et al., 2021).

Symptomatic voice therapy alone is not usually enough to resolve the PVD-related dysphonia or aphonia, and psychological support to supplement our work may be required to address the deeper distress the client is experiencing (Tezcaner et al., 2019). This may come from counselling, a clinical psychologist or psychiatric services if the client is already known to them. Cognitive behavioural therapy (CBT) is emerging as a valuable complement to traditional voice therapy (Gray et al., in press) but needs to be provided by trained CBT professionals and Tip 47 differentiates the roles of the difference health professionals supporting mental well-being. You should recognise the limits of your scope of practice and discuss any onward referral so clients understand why wider support is being recommended and you have their consent to make the referral.

Looking after the therapist's well-being

All tender conversations are confidential unless your client has given permission to share specific details with other health professionals and with two other exceptions – firstly, when what you hear suggests the client is at risk of harm or harming others and you need to share information to protect your client or others and secondly, when you discuss your experiences as part of formal supervision. Being human is, by its very nature, complex, and clients may divulge details unexpectedly, which not only changes your management plan but challenges our practice. Therapists working at all levels of expertise should have access to professional support. For student SLTs, your supervising therapist will be able to provide this, newly qualified practitioners are likely to have a mentor and even the most experienced therapists should have access to clinical supervision.

TIP 29 – VOCAL FOLD NODULES

> *Typical voice quality*: rough and breathy. The nodules distort the straight edge on the vocal folds which causes roughness, and breathiness arises from the incomplete closure due to the presence of nodules.
> *Common causes*: overuse and poor voice production.
> *Treatment*: direct and indirect voice therapy with a focus on reducing phonotraumatic behaviours. As the nodules resolve, the voice quality should improve unless the client has a further period of vocally damaging behaviours resulting in repeated, or extended, vocal deterioration.

Do you remember Bastian and Thomas' (2016) concept of the vocal overdoer in Tip 15? Clients with nodules are typically the overdoers. They usually have high amounts of voice use with high intensity, which contributes to long-distance doses, heavy phonatory load, and high cycle doses (Assad et al., 2017). They are also often female, young, and someone who talks a lot for a living or who enjoys talking with others, and if we asked them to rate themselves on a 0–10 scale of chattiness amongst their friends, they might opt for the higher ratings, without full awareness of just how much they are using their voice or the impact of vocally demanding situations. Listeners may comment that they sound like "they've had a good night out" and some clients believe the breathy quality to be sexy but you should remind them that this voice quality reflects damage. Without change, nodules will worsen and be more difficult to reduce.

Often nodules are attributed to vocal misuse or abuse, and although there can indeed be phonotraumatic behaviours, using such negative and non-complementary language may reduce clients' sense of self-efficacy (Gillespie & Verdolini Abbott, 2011) so we should be careful with how we describe the likely cause of the nodules. Terminology aside, voice conservation will be a key focus of your management plan, working with your client to identify opportunities throughout the day as shorter, frequent periods of rest are more effective than one long rest at the end of the day. Although clients may think there is no scope for rest, particularly if their work is vocally demanding, it is usually possible to find small periods of time through collaborative discussion. For instance, teachers can rest their voice by not chatting to colleagues during break time (which may mean they don't go to the staff room if it is too tempting to socialise), fitness instructors can rest their voice by not speaking between classes, and students can rest their voice by reducing chatter between classes or when socialising.

Following advice about voice rest should bring about voice improvement fairly quickly if overuse is one of few contributing factors to the dysphonia. From experience, there can be an audible improvement within a couple of weeks of starting to increase rest periods, though it takes longer before resolution of the nodules is seen on laryngeal evaluation. Indeed, the voice may be perceptually normal or only mildly dysphonic while remnant nodules may exist (Jo et al., 2021). An improving voice should reassure clients that their investment in voice conservation is effective and may foster continued commitment to improved vocal care as they must not become complacent. The heterogeneous nature of our voices and individualised vocal demands means there isn't a definitive answer to the question of how much voice rest is enough but think of it this way: just as we wouldn't go on a long day's hike without pausing for lunch or a moment to enjoy the view after a burst of uphill exertion, our clients also benefit from vocal pit-stops throughout the day and after periods of vocal exertion. Where voice rest is challenging to achieve, return to Tip 4 for a reminder on change and Tip 12 for managing slower progress. If poor voice production technique is also contributing, modification of this will also be required before feeling and hearing greater benefit.

In the Introduction, I mentioned a university friend who was diagnosed with vocal fold nodules. She was a committed goalkeeper in our hockey club, shouting instructions to the rest of the team from her perfect visual position at the back of the field. She demonstrated similar commitment to socialising and, at the time, also smoked occasionally. Knowing what I was studying, she shared her diagnosis but I didn't quite know what to say when she informed me she'd been told not to drink, smoke, or shout and hadn't any intention of following this advice, being proud of what was branded "Tour Voice"! Talking to her about it now, she acknowledges that the SLT advice wasn't compatible with the lifestyle she wanted to lead at the time but studying overseas later in her degree and working in a non-vocally demanding job post-graduation allowed her voice to heal over time and it is now used sensibly and without dysphonia. I also recall a colleague booking a client with vocal fold nodules for 4 o'clock on a Friday afternoon which was outside of my colleague's usual appointment schedule timetable but accommodated the client's working pattern. Unfortunately the client failed to attend but was spotted an hour later standing on a bench in a bar enjoying after-work drinks! It is therefore important you have a full picture of voice use, using probing questions to understand your client's motivations for therapy, reasons for attending, and hindrances to practice. Behlau et al.'s (in press) coaching questions, mentioned in Tips 5 and 6, are of relevance here too.

You may now be wondering how you recommend voice rest without suggesting the client doesn't have any fun. It can be helpful to see the voice like a bank account where each speaking situation withdraws some "vocal currency". If you are a student, you may withdraw more vocal cash on placement days than when on campus where you have breaks between classes and at least some of your time in class will be listening to others. Whether the withdrawals are regular or infrequent, we each need to ensure we're not vocally overdrawn at any point of the day or week.

Table 1 provides an example of voice use across a day and self-development activity 20 encourages you to complete your own record of this.

In this example I never become vocally overdrawn, although you can see my voice bank gradually decrease. Investing in voice rest on my return commute and not speaking while

Table 1 A sample summary of voice use.

Time of day	Monday	Vocal "cash" used	Vocal cash remaining
AM	Starting balance		100
	Breakfast conversation with family	−10	90
	Commute to work, singing along to two gentle songs	−5	85
	Meeting to discuss waiting list with colleagues	−10	75
	Client 1 (initial case history)	−10	65
	15 minutes to write up notes	+5	70
	Client 2 (breathing and relaxation session)	−5	65
	15 minutes to write up notes	+5	70
	1 hour of review phone calls + writing up of notes	−5	65
PM	30 minutes' lunch break with colleagues.	−10	55
	Client 3 (counselling focused, lots of active listening)	−5	50
	15 minutes to write up notes	+5	55
	Client 4 (projection practice with a fitness instructor including lots of demonstration)	−15	40
	15 minutes to write up notes	+5	45
	Client 5 (experimentation of safe use of character voices with a primary teacher)	−15	30
	15 minutes to write up notes	+5	35
	Silent commute home – voice tired!	+20	55

(*continued*)

Table 1 Cont.

Time of day	Monday	Vocal "cash" used	Vocal cash remaining
	Quiet time while getting ready for dinner with friends	+10	65
	Quick phone call with hard-of-hearing relative	–5	60
	Dinner with friends – chatty as I haven't seen them for a while!	–25	35
	Natural voice rest overnight	+ lots!	

I write my case notes ensures I don't reach a "danger zone" of having no vocal funds at all. However, if I was to go to a festival for five days and unrealistically attempt to compete with the amplified singers' voices, I would probably run out of voice funds quickly and develop hoarseness.

SELF-DEVELOPMENT ACTIVITY 20 – COMPLETING YOUR OWN VOICE DIARY

To extend your reflections from self-development activity 4 about your own voice care, complete a voice diary for a typical day.

- How close to being vocally overdrawn are you?
- Could you add in any additional opportunities for voice rest to reduce this risk?

Now complete it for a day or an event during which you think you will find it more difficult to conserve your voice.

- What have you learnt from these reflections?

If the self-development activity above revealed vocally harmful behaviours, perhaps you can pay attention! If you have a reluctance to change your practices, can you identify what contributes to that in the context of your role to encourage others to be more careful with their voice? If you don't relate to the vocally harmful behaviours and do take good care of your voice, well done! You can empathise with your clients about the challenges of staying on top of good voice care but show it is possible to minimise phonotraumatic habits without this requiring a significant withdrawal from social interactions.

Surgical intervention

Clients may enquire about surgery if they have misunderstood celebrity surgery for polyps as also being relevant for nodules, or if they have seen films such as Pitch Perfect which suggest this is a typical route for management. Internationally there are different surgical attitudes but this is often reserved for nodules unlikely to resolve with voice conservation and improved speaking or singing technique. If the underlying factors contributing to the nodules are not addressed, the nodules can reform and, as scar tissue arising from surgery has a negative impact on the voice, unless this is the only solution to the problem, surgery is usually avoided.

TIP 30 – REINKE'S OEDEMA

> *Typical voice quality*: rough, deepened pitch, and possible compensatory strain.
> *Common causes*: smoking, poor voice production technique.
> *Treatment*: direct and indirect voice therapy, usually with a focus on smoking cessation.

Although fluid can accumulate in Reinke's space through misuse of the voice, it typically occurs due to smoking. This fullness in the vocal folds, visible on EEL, contributes to a deeper pitch, which is why female smokers may be mistaken for male speakers if there are no visual cues as to the speaker's gender. The swelling removes the straight edge of the vocal folds, contributing to a rough quality, and speakers may also add in muscular tension to compensate for the emerging hoarseness.

Indirect therapy

The focus of vocal care advice should be smoking cessation, not only to reduce the oedema but to reduce a future risk of laryngeal cancer. Although Reinke's oedema and cancer are not directly linked, clients should be aware that Reinke's oedema doesn't prevent subsequent development of abnormal cells, and Tip 48 provides contact details for national smoking cessation associations. Unlike vocal fold nodules where voice improvement can be heard relatively quickly with dedicated voice care, improvement in clients with Reinke's oedema is much more gradual. This slower progress can be less motivating and clients may go through several cycles of trying to make change before developing new habits (Tip 4). Reiterating that they are investing in their overall health, as well as investing in their voice, may encourage smoking cessation.

If you are unsure how to recommend someone stops smoking, I encourage you write a script and practise this with family members or friends. Use your developing skills in tender conversations (Tip 7) to listen to the challenges that your client may be experiencing in giving up smoking and explain the importance of this with sensitivity. Some clients may have been smoking for decades, possibly since their teenage years, and may not want to give up this pleasure, others may see stopping a longstanding habit as an impossibility, and others may resist the feeling of being told what to do. A simple way of finding out about the client's relationship with smoking is to make reference to this when you outline your forward plan: *"you said earlier that you've smoked since you were X years/for a long time/because you're feeling stressed at the moment, and I can understand it's hard to break a habit but we know smoking is not good for the voice. It can cause swelling of the vocal folds which leads to a rough and deeper voice (if the client already has evidence of laryngeal changes, such as Reinke's oedema, you can add that in too) and I know my Ear, Nose and Throat colleagues are always worried that smoking can lead to more worrying changes in the voice box such as cancer. So this doesn't have a further impact on your voice, I'm going to recommend that you stop smoking, and I can support you to do this. What do you think about giving up?"*

Direct therapy

If your client has developed secondary muscle tension dysphonia in response to Reinke's-related hoarseness, therapy to address voice production is also advised and you can plan therapy with Tip 27 in mind.

Surgical intervention

Occasionally, where the oedema is so great that it could compromise the client's airway and hinder respiration, a surgical decision is taken to drain the fluid through mucosal incision, microdebrider (the use of a rotating blade to "shave" the affected tissues), or carbon dioxide laser (Khodeir et al., 2021). Where surgery is not essential to maintain a patent airway but is offered by the surgeon to improve the voice, an important consideration is whether your client will return to smoking post-surgery – just like vocal fold nodules, there is little benefit to removing the pathology if the controllable contributing factors continue. We also need to note that even where surgical intervention is recommended and smoking stops, the voice may not return to a normal quality (Martins et al., 2017).

TIP 31 – GRANULOMAS

> *Typical voice quality*: rough with possible breathiness if the granuloma prevents complete vocal fold closure. The voice may fatigue easily and these symptoms may also be accompanied by a globus sensation and pain.
>
> *Common causes*: irritation from reflux, phonotrauma, and laryngeal trauma from intubation. The pathology can be unilateral or bilateral.
>
> *Treatment*: direct and indirect voice therapy.

Indirect therapy

Your input will ensure clients are maintaining good vocal hygiene and, where anti-reflux medication is prescribed by either the client's GP or ENT consultant, you will supplement this with reflux-reducing advice such as avoiding spicy, acidic, and processed foods, alcohol, caffeine, and eating late at night.

Direct therapy

Particularly where phonotrauma has been the cause of laryngeal granuloma(s), your therapy will address voice production, influenced by your assessment findings and taking into consideration your client's vocal demands. Therapy can overlap with that for functional voice disorder in Tip 27 if the voice production technique is less than optimal and may also be similar to vocal fold nodules in Tip 29 if there have been vocally harmful behaviours.

If intubation or reflux are the main precipitating factors for the granuloma, your input is unlikely to be extensive though you may hear of the outcome of medical intervention if your client attends a joint ENT-SLT Voice Clinic for review.

Surgical intervention

Although surgical removal may be necessary if the granuloma is obstructing the airway, this intervention risks recurrence and therefore conservative treatment combining anti-reflux treatment with voice therapy is usually the first line of defence.

TIP 32 – VOCAL FOLD PALSIES

> *Typical voice quality*: dependent on the position of the palsied vocal fold, the speaking voice will sound near normal or breathy.
>
> *Common causes*: most usually caused by a lesion of the recurrent laryngeal nerve from trauma, surgery, or pressure on the nerve, with a small number of superior laryngeal nerve lesions from trauma. In most cases the palsy is unilateral.
>
> *Treatment*: direct and indirect voice therapy with a focus on vocal strengthening. Bulk injection for abducted palsies and surgical intervention where respiratory function is hindered by an adducted position of the palsied vocal fold(s). Swallowing assessment may also be required where an abducted palsy reduces airway protection and places your client at risk of aspiration.

Endoscopic evaluation of the larynx will reveal whether a vocal fold palsy (VFP) is sitting in an abducted position or an adducted position, and each influences respiration and phonation in different ways. *Ab*ducted means it is sitting away from the midline and if *ad*ducted, it is sitting towards the midline. Figure 10a represents normal vocal fold positions at rest and on phonation for context, Figure 10b shows the impact of a left *ab*ducted vocal fold palsy (VFP) on respiration and phonation by comparison, and Figure 10c shows the impact of a left *ad*ducted VFP on respiration and phonation. The same impacts occur in mirror image for a right VFP depending on whether it sits in an abducted or adducted position.

Indirect therapy

Although there may be a clear cause-and-effect for the VFP, don't forget to ask your client the usual questions about vocal health and then educate them as required. The British Voice

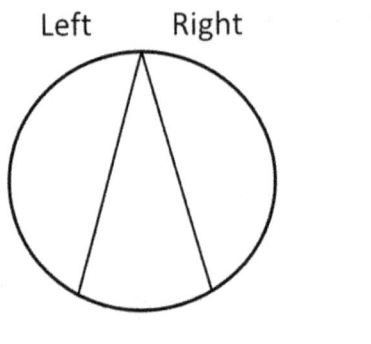
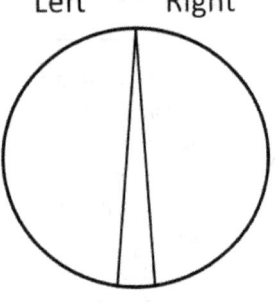

Figure 10a Normal vocal fold position at rest and on phonation

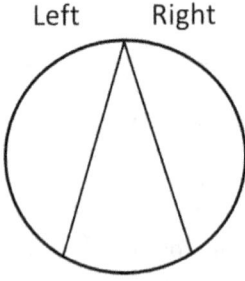
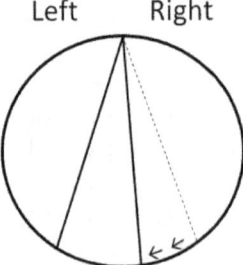

Left *ab*ducted VFP
- at rest

Left *ab*ducted VFP
- on phonation

Little impact as respiration is not impeded and phonation is not being attempted.

Because the palsied vocal fold sits *away* from the midline, the gap between the vocal folds leads to a breathy voice quality from the extra air escape.

Figure 10b Impact of a left abducted VFP at rest and on phonation

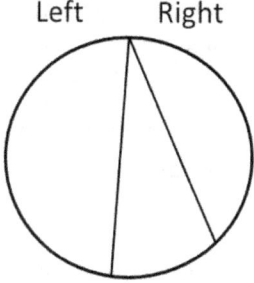 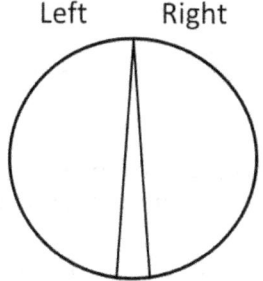

Left adducted VFP
- at rest

Left adducted VFP
- on phonation

The reduced airway space may impact little on respiration at rest but breathing may be more difficult on exertion.

Because the palsied vocal fold sits *near* the midline the vocal folds are close on phonation which contributes to a clearer voice quality.

Figure 10c Impact of a left adducted VFP at rest and on phonation

Association has produced a factsheet to help you and your clients understand VFP and the link is at the end of this chapter.

Direct therapy

For clients with temporary nerve damage there will be spontaneous recovery of the voice within three to nine months, though this can be accelerated by therapy aiming to strengthen the palsied vocal fold. From your reading of the management chapter and your understanding of primary and secondary muscle tension dysphonia, you should have a sense that therapy often focuses on reducing effort in speaking. Therapy to aid recovery from a vocal fold palsy departs from this common thread in that it asks clients to use greater effort to strengthen the muscles around the vocal folds and develop compensation for the palsy.

This needs to be balanced with exercises which prevent the build-up of tension and strain from using greater effort. Try self-development activity 21 to experience this yourself.

> **SELF-DEVELOPMENT ACTIVITY 21 – VOCAL FOLD STRENGTHENING EXERCISES**
>
> Sit on a chair and hold on to the edges of the seat and pull up the seat towards you. Hold for three seconds and then release. What do you notice?
>
> Now, try a yawn as you've done in Tip 25. What are you aware of around your neck in comparison with the task above? If you're not sure what you notice, alternate between these movements two or three times.
>
> When you pull up on the chair, the vocal folds meet together in the same valving manoeuvre as if we were lifting something heavy. The temporary stop to your breath is then released as you let go of the seat. The valving action develops strength and then the yawn releases tension so the focus is on developing strength, not strain.

Your case history data should also include whether the client has any swallowing difficulties. Palsied vocal folds sitting in an abducted position result in incomplete airway protection during swallowing and increase the risk of aspiration – they also contribute to a weaker cough from reduced glottic pressure so there is compromised ability to clear the airway of any penetrated saliva, food, or drink.

Surgical intervention

Surgical intervention will be influenced by the position of the palsied vocal fold, balancing the relative risks of breathing and voice (de Almeida et al., in press). Where an abducted vocal fold palsy significantly compromises phonation or safe swallowing, injection laryngoplasty can increase the volume of, and medialise, the paralysed vocal fold to reduce the glottic gap. This is done only when there is strong evidence of no possible recovery in the affected vocal fold as there is a risk of an occluded airway and respiratory complications should the treated vocal fold move towards the midline after intervention. Arytenoidectomy and cordotomy aim to enlarge the airway where respiration is hindered but this brings risks of granuloma formation, scarring, and poor voice quality.

For vocal fold palsies caused by pressure on the recurrent laryngeal nerve from a tumour, surgical removal or de-bulking of the tumour can alleviate some of the dysphonia but cancer diagnoses may understandably be a more pressing concern and priority for health treatment than voice therapy.

TIP 33 – UPPER AIRWAY DISORDERS

Although upper airway voice disorders (UADs) can co-exist with, or be misdiagnosed as, respiratory disorders, the symptoms are located around the throat rather than the lungs. These conditions require liaison with respiratory physicians, respiratory physiotherapists, and possibly clinical psychologists in addition to the usual liaison with our ENT colleagues. Complementing their position paper on the management of UADs, the RCSLT has produced a useful factsheet and the link is in the reference list.

Chronic cough

Arising from irritation in the larynx, chronic cough is characterised by a dry cough which persists for more than eight weeks. Medical assessment is required before clients attend SLT to discount possible causes such as a respiratory infection or disease, heart problems, a reaction to medication, postnasal drip, or reflux. It can be related to asthma but can also occur in isolation from a lung condition. Recent research suggests there may also be an influence from laryngeal sensitivity (Sundar et al., 2021) and an impairment in cough inhibition.

Tip 14 reminded you of the importance of a holistic approach to voice and we also consider chronic cough from a holistic perspective. We aim to understand the frequency and duration of the cough, the possible triggers, the associated sensations, and the impact. Shembel et al.'s (2013) 10-item Cough Severity Index asks clients to rate the frequency and impact of their symptoms and it can be used over time to monitor change and act as an outcome measure.

In Tip 29 we considered the cyclical nature of throat clearing, and chronic cough can also be cyclical, with coughing giving rise to vocal fold irritation, more coughing, and a subsequent risk of vocal fold pathology if left untreated. To discourage coughing, as we discourage throat clearing, clients are advised to take a sip of water, swallow, and repeat until the desire to cough subsides. We will also use voice training to reduce irritation of the larynx and our skills in tender conversations

(Tip 7) to support clients in coping with this condition. Cough suppressant strategies should not be advised until a diagnosis of chronic cough is confirmed in case this masks an underlying pathology.

Inducible laryngeal obstruction (ILO)

Defined as "an inappropriate, transient, reversible narrowing of the larynx in response to external triggers" (Halvorsen et al., 2017, p. 1), ILO was previously known more broadly as vocal fold dysfunction. It is characterised by a choking sensation and wheeze, triggered by exercise, chemicals, odours (such as strong perfume or spices), stress, reflux, and specific voice tasks. At its worst, unmanaged breathlessness arising from an obstructed airflow may prompt a call for emergency medical help. Halvorsen et al. (2017) present possible neural and mechanical causes for ILO but our understanding of this condition is still growing. A possible psychological cause has been both proposed and discounted, and the psychological panic is more widely understood as a response to the respiratory distress rather than a cause of it. Like chronic cough, it is diagnosed by a multidisciplinary team.

Although we sometimes talk of needing to "catch our breath", this phrasing suggests management of inhalations but this is harder to do than working with our exhalations. Encouraging clients to breathe out helps reset the breath because once we exhale, our lungs automatically attempt to replenish the breath so the cycle is gently reset. Understandably, clients may panic during the onset of breathing difficulties, particularly if ILO has yet to be diagnosed, but the body tension and respiratory disruption associated with panic unfortunately compound the difficulty.

To increase laryngeal control and as an emergency release strategy clients should practise this three-step response:

- sniff in
- blow out as if blowing out a candle (short blow)
- blow out as if blowing into a balloon (long blow)

Like chronic cough, our indirect intervention will draw on tender conversation skills as we listen empathically and actively to our clients' concerns, respond to their distress, and consider their stress if this is a contributing factor. If the triggers for our clients' ILO can reasonably be avoided, we will also suggest they avoid exposure, with recognition that this may not always be possible in public places.

TIP 34 – PRESBYPHONIA

> *Typical voice quality*: weaker, fatiguing voice.
> *Common causes*: vocal fold atrophy and bowing of the vocal folds, leading to incomplete glottic closure.
> *Treatment*: direct and indirect voice therapy to optimise current vocal fold function with possible guidance around increasing vocal load.

Presbyphonia describes age-related voice difficulties – just as older adults notice changes in mobility and general upper body strength, changes to the laryngeal musculature as part of the normal ageing process contribute to a weaker voice. If this is concomitant with reduced vocal use, there is a cumulative effect of musculature changes leading to function changes, and avoidance of conversation from the function changes leads to further changes in musculature. Some clients with presbyphonia who have been professional voice users hypothesise that they've "worn out" their voices with high vocal demands when they were working but there is no evidence at present to suggest a direct causal link.

In Tip 15 we considered the concept of vocal overdoers and underdoers. Although some clients with presbyphonia may use their voices regularly during social engagements with friends or meetings of voluntary committees, others will be vocal underdoers (Ziegler & Hapner, 2020), influenced by not working, being widowed, living alone, or other health issues which limit social engagement. Lower voice use may contribute to lower self-rated impairment (Ebersole et al., 2017) and, coupled with reassurance at the lack of malignancy and a lack of significant symptoms some clients may decline the offer of therapy. Conversely others will be keen for input to improve their voice, based on frustration at voice change and poorer function in the voice (Young, 2020).

Direct therapy

Unlike our clients with vocal fold nodules who are advised to rest their voices, clients with vocal fold atrophy, or presbylaryngis, will be encouraged to use them on a "use it or lose it" basis.

Spending a day without much voice use and then entering a speaking-heavy situation is the equivalent of transitioning between a rest and a sprint for our presbyphonic clients, so it is important to limber up the vocal system. Our advice will include gentle warm up exercises (Tip 45), particularly prior to social engagements or telephone calls where there is otherwise a long period of low voice use. If health conditions or personal circumstances prevent clients from attending regular SLT appointments to practise warm-up exercises, an alternative option is to keep the voice ticking over through gentle talking. This can easily be done through a commentary of what's going on around them (e.g. "it's sunny outside today so I'll hang out the washing and then I'll make a cup of tea. I'm looking forward to meeting my sister later for a chat and telling her about my holiday"). The content doesn't matter so much as the fact there is gentle voice use.

Occurring alongside vocal fold atrophy may be generalised weakness in the respiratory system, either age-related or due to specific respiratory diagnoses, and this will influence expiration control, aerodynamic power, and the length of utterances. Other vocal or upper body structures may be engaged to compensate and whilst this hyperfunction may maintain adequate airflow resistance, it reduces vocal fold pliability (Desjardins et al., 2022) and increases tension. Your therapy plan will therefore need to take account of any maladaptive strategies and you can approach this from a functional perspective (Tip 27).

Incomplete glottic closure from the bowed shape of the vocal folds leads speakers to run out of breath more quickly in conversation than a speaker whose vocal folds fully adduct. In this case, therapy should consider shortening the utterances and increasing the frequency of top-up breaths so adequate breath support is maintained, as in Tip 25.

Unfortunately, traditional exercises aiming to increase breath support are unlikely to be sufficiently intensive to change the underlying respiratory system. Instead a combination of voice therapy with Respiratory Muscle Strength Training (RMST) can increase respiratory strength and reduce hyperfunction (Desjardins et al., 2022), with improvement noted on self-rating scores (Belafsky et al., in press).

Co-morbid difficulties

Hearing loss isn't directly related to presbyphonia but can co-occur and, whilst motivation for therapy may remain, hearing difficulties can hinder the progression of therapy (Park et al., in press). Remember clients need to develop their own sensory awareness of voice production (Tip 23) and if hearing is impaired, clients may not hear your modelling and may find self-monitoring difficult.

Alternatively, if your client doesn't have their own hearing difficulties, they may be living with someone who does. In this case you will also need to incorporate safe projection in your therapy plan and identify strategies to reduce the impact of hearing difficulties on two-way communication. Advice may include turning off background noise so your client's voice can be heard without strain, and ensuring the speaker and listener are facing each other for supplementary facial cues, lip reading and gesture. Where any client is in regular contact with someone with hearing difficulties, do check whether hearing aids are a) used and b) effective. Do not assume that both are true!

TIP 35 – SPASMODIC DYSPHONIA

> *Typical voice quality*: strained and strangled with intermittent voice breaks for adductor spasmodic dysphonia. Breathy with intermittent voice breaks for abductor spasmodic dysphonia.
> *Common causes*: neurological, though the underlying cause of the neurological differences is not yet fully understood.
> *Treatment*: direct and indirect voice therapy alongside botulinum toxin injection.

Spasmodic dysphonia (SD) takes three forms: adductor spasmodic dysphonia (AdSD) as the most common subtype, abductor spasmodic dysphonia (AbSD), and mixed spasmodic dysphonia. The involuntary muscle spasms only occur during phonation. It is rare and usually affects females starting in their 40s.

Although there is agreement that SD is a neurological condition, research continues to investigate what underlies the neurological differences in this acquired voice disorder. Hintze et al.'s (2017) review suggests that a family history of neurological disorders, recent viral illness and heavy voice use contribute to the development of SD and this is extended by Vanderaa and Vinney (in press) who consider laryngeal hypersensitivity and long-term sequelae from upper respiratory tract infections to be contributing factors.

Surgical intervention

As an incurable condition, medical management focuses on symptom relief through intramuscular botulinum toxin injections. Performed while the client is awake, these cause flaccid paralysis of the muscles which can lead to good temporary reduction of the spasms but repeated injections are usually needed to maintain the impact (Stachler et al., 2018) and the timeframe for these is personalised to the individual client (Yorkston et al., 2021). Although quality of life (QoL) for clients with AdSD is often improved through botulinum toxin injection, most don't reach normal QoL levels, which may be due to both the voice quality and chronic nature of SD (Faham et al., 2021).

Speech and language therapy intervention

Alongside botulinum toxin as the surgical solution, we are in the ideal position to listen to the client's concerns and the impact of SD since we know it can cause significant disruption to a client's social participation and workplace productivity (Meyer et al., 2021). Clients may appreciate the benefits of injection and how this limits deterioration but this doesn't fully mitigate against withdrawal from conversations (Yorkston et al., 2021). For all client groups, we want our clients to have a voice and feel heard, so avoiding conversation isn't a healthy long-term strategy, even if we can understand it as a logical short-term solution when clients are experiencing communication difficulty. Our role in therapy, using our tender conversation skills (Tip 7) will be to support the client to maintain their contributions in conversation and live positively with this chronic condition.

TIP 36 – PREPARING FOR SURGERY

For clients requiring surgical intervention to improve their voice as in Tips 37, 38, and 39, SLT input will be wrapped round the date of surgery with pre-operative voice education, post-operative voice rest, and post-operative voice therapy, the sequence of which is in Figure 11.

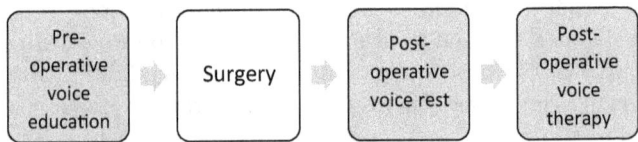

Figure 11   The three stages of SLT intervention for surgical voice clients

Pre-operative voice education

Post-operative voice care needs to come before surgery as it's too late to wait until the first SLT appointment after the operation – voice care starts from the moment your client wakes up from anaesthesia. Where vocal irritants and phonotraumatic behaviours have contributed to the lesion under surgical management, these should be addressed pre-surgery with the same guidance reiterated post-surgery (White & Carding, 2020). Pre-operative counsel will also include information about post-operative voice rest and how, and when, the client should start using their voice again. This education prepares the client for what to expect around surgery and gives warning about the importance of voice rest in case changes to work or family commitments are required. For some clients, pre-operative voice therapy may even prevent the need for surgery.

Post-operative voice rest

Voice rest is imperative after surgery. Complete voice rest (CVR) occurs in the acute post-operative period and requires an alternative means of communication, such as writing, alongside a ban on any whispering or throat clearing. It is followed by relative voice rest (RVR) during which there should still be no traumatic vocal behaviours such as shouting or singing and voice use is limited to essential talking only. Unfortunately, the research is inconclusive regarding the optimal duration of the voice rest with an average of four to five days' CVR recommended in a European study (Rihkanen & Geneid, 2019) and one to seven days' CVR, dependent on pathology, recommended in a US study (Joshi & Johns, 2018). Kaneko et al.'s (2017) work suggests that clients resting their voice for three days achieved better long-term outcomes than those resting their voice for seven days, and there is certainly a balance to be struck between wound healing and nurturing early epithelium remobilisation. In the absence of clear and agreed guidelines you need to follow the recommendations given by your client's ENT consultant.

To be prepared for written communication immediately after their operation, clients should take pen and paper or a mobile phone to the hospital, writing down any specific questions they have for medical, nursing, or SLT teams in advance. Some SLT departments have pre-printed phrases including statements around how clients are feeling (e.g. I'm in pain) or questions about their care (e.g. can I go to the hospital shop?). Not so long ago, when telephones were limited to making calls clients would have been more isolated from their social network during CVR but with a wealth of communication apps and social media outlets now available, you can reassure clients that they can still connect with family and friends while they have total voice rest. If your client is particularly talkative and likely to find voice rest difficult, it would be worth encouraging them to experiment with periods of no voice use, as in self-development activity 5, prior to having to do this when it matters.

Beyond their short hospital admission, you will need to consider your client's working demands as CVR and RVR guidance applies to all environments. If there are expectations of verbal communication in an office environment, even if those are purely social, clients may need to explore working from home or a period of sick leave, though sick leave recommendations have ranged widely from 0 to 35 days (Rihkanen & Geneid, 2019)! As you will see in Tip 49, employers have a legal duty to support clients with any condition that makes their job more difficult, and this includes modifying occupational duties during periods of voice rest and voice restoration. An operation date will largely depend on the surgeon's schedule but where there is a choice of date, opting for a day nearer to the client's typical days off reduces the need for sick leave. Clients are not legally obliged to do this but some aim to construe this plan if they have had repeated surgical procedures, each with accompanying periods of sick leave, as for clients with recurrent laryngeal papillomas. There can be guilt around being off work if colleagues are required to cover and not all employment comes with paid sick leave.

Once the recommended period of complete voice rest has passed, RVR reintroduces low amounts of gentle voice use. This can be as simple as a "good morning" greeting to a family member or housemate, a short response when asked how they are feeling or a question about what to have for lunch but the overall sentiment at this stage is avoiding long conversations, projection, and singing.

Post-operative voice therapy

Remembering not to schedule an appointment for the first week post-op when your client is not speaking or is limiting their conversation, you will want to review your client's voice after surgery through repeated acoustic-perceptual assessment, observation of voice production style, and discussion regarding the impact of surgery for your client. If therapy is required to address voice difficulties unrelated to the pathology, you should plan this according to your client's needs (Tip 19).

White et al.'s (in press) systematic review of pre- and postoperative voice therapy intervention intended to compile a surgical rehabilitation programme based on the available evidence but heterogeneity of clients, a lack of information around the timing, intensity, and content of intervention, and high variability across the intervention provided or outcome measurement prevent that currently. As with research around the optimal duration of CVR and RVR, further work is needed to develop a robust intervention framework for surgical voice clients but in upholding person-centredness and evidence-based practice in our care, any intervention should be personalised to the client.

TIP 37 – LARYNGEAL PAPILLOMA

> *Typical voice quality*: rough from the pathology interfering with the straight edge of the vocal folds. There may be additional strain from maladaptive voice production in response to the roughness. Deterioration in voice quality can continue between laryngeal assessment and the day of surgery as the wart-like growths continue to spread.
>
> *Common causes*: the underlying cause is the human papilloma virus but it is not known why this specifically develops into laryngeal papillomas for some people.
>
> *Treatment*: surgical intervention to remove the papillomatous tissue with direct and indirect voice therapy. Repeated surgical intervention and therapy blocks may be required with papilloma regrowth.

Surgical intervention

Left untreated, papillomatous tissue may obstruct the airway so this is removed through a microdebrider, laser, or very fine surgical instruments, and decisions regarding the surgical method will be determined by local practice and the extent of the lesion. A key aim of surgery will be to preserve the vocal folds' delicate layers and particular care will be taken when operating bilaterally near the anterior commissure to prevent the formation of a laryngeal web from scar tissue. Some surgeons may operate separately on each vocal fold where there is bilateral papilloma growth.

Adjuvant intervention via drug injection into the vocal fold may be done at the time of surgery which aims to control disease progression, rather than cure it. A consensus on the effectiveness of different drugs, which currently include bevacizumab (common name: Avastin), cidofovir (common name: Vistide), and Gardasil, is difficult due to the high variability in how papillomas progress for each client (Ballestas et al., 2021).

For some clients, one surgical intervention is sufficient to remove the papillomatous tissue but many need repeated surgical procedures, sometimes within the same year and sometimes over several years before regrowth stops. Just as we don't have evidence for what precipitates the development of laryngeal papillomas, we also don't yet know why they suddenly stop growing. Reassuringly, there may not be a cumulative negative effect on voice quality from repeated surgery (Parker et al., 2020) though further evidence is needed to be very certain about this.

Direct therapy

From clinical experience, the pattern of papilloma regrowth for some clients can seem to coincide with periods of increased client stress. There is no published literature regarding this but, whether stress is a factor in regrowth or not, living with a variable and unpredictable condition is inherently a stressful experience and therefore a degree of anxiety is to be expected. The impact of a potentially chronic condition can permeate work, home, and personal lives so we should call on our tender conversation skills (Tip 7) to support our clients.

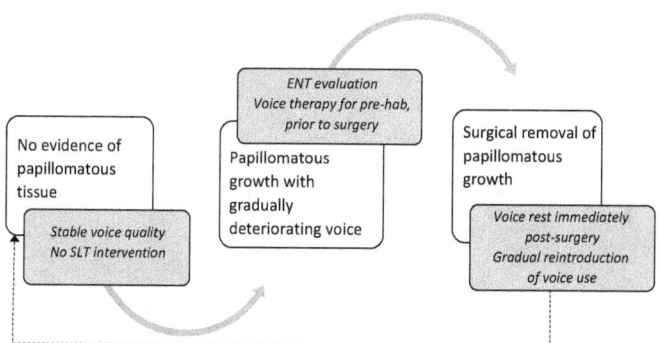

Figure 12 A cycle of SLT input in relation to papilloma growth

Our direct involvement with this client group will follow the pathway in the previous tip, with education provided pre-therapy and voice therapy provided after voice rest has concluded. Voice therapy exercises will be tailored to the most pressing concern for the client but will certainly aim to prevent the development of secondary muscle tension dysphonia (Tip 27). Where repeated surgical procedures are needed, clients may also attend for repeated SLT intervention, as in Figure 12.

TIP 38 – VOCAL FOLD POLYPS

> *Typical voice quality*: rough from the pathology interfering in smooth vocal fold movement, and breathiness if the site of the polyp limits vocal fold closure. There may be additional strain from maladaptive voice production in response to the dysphonia.
> *Common causes*: short-term phonotrauma (unilateral polyp), reflux or chronic inhalation of irritants such as industrial fumes (bilateral polyps).
> *Treatment*: direct and indirect voice therapy with possible surgery.

Unlike vocal fold nodules which develop over time, vocal fold polyps can develop through short-term phonotrauma such as shouting and cheering at a sporting event. They differ from papillomas in that polyps do not increase in size between laryngeal assessment and surgery so the voice quality heard at initial assessment will be consistent until the lesion is removed.

Complete resolution of smaller and more recently developed polyps is possible with conservative voice therapy alone (Nakagawa et al., 2012; Zhuge et al., 2016), particularly for female clients (Nakagawa et al., 2012; Lee et al., 2017). We still need large-scale studies for a clear statement about the influence of the size and shape of a polyp on voice quality though, as a bigger polyp does not necessarily mean greater severity of dysphonia given the heterogeneous nature of our voices (Öcal et al., 2020). There may be greater impact from a small polyp for a client reliant on their voice for work compared with a client with a larger polyp but fewer vocal demands.

Where surgery is required, the client should be provided with pre-operative advice as in Tip 36 and consideration given to post-operative voice therapy to address any maladaptive voice production and vocal care in general.

TIP 39 – VOCAL FOLD CYSTS

Typical voice quality: rough if the cyst interferes with smooth vibration and breathy if the vocal folds are unable to vibrate closely together. This will depend on the location of the cyst.

Common causes: mucous retention cysts are caused by a mucus-producing gland becoming blocked to form a sac of fluid or semi-solid material. Epidermoid cysts are usually longstanding and may only be identified when the client's vocal demands increase and the impact of a cyst is observed. Unlike other vocal fold lesions, cysts are not associated with phonotrauma.

Treatment: surgical intervention. If secondary muscle tension dysphonia has developed in response to the dysphonia, direct and indirect voice therapy may be helpful.

In Tip 2, I cited work by Kristie Knickerbocker and colleagues which sought to understand vocal load. Kristie is an American speech and language pathologist whose experience of a vocal fold cyst changed her career path from aspiring singer to therapist and her account of voice difficulties from a professional's perspective is in Hutchins (2018).

There may be little for the SLT to do for a client with a cyst, unless they are a professional voice user who has developed secondary muscle tension dysphonia in response to cyst-related voice difficulties and you can exploit this opportunity to educate them more broadly about safe voice use.

REFERENCES

Aghadoost, S., Jalaie, S., Khatoonabadi, A. R., Dabirmoghaddam, P. & Khoddami, S. M. (2020) A Study of Vocal Facilitating Techniques Compared to Manual Circumlaryngeal Therapy in Teachers with Muscle Tension Dysphonia.

Journal of Voice 34 (6) 963.e11–963.e21 https://doi.org/10.1016/j.jvoice.2019.06.002

Assad, J. P., de castro Magalhães, Santos, J. N. & Gama, A. C. C. (2017) Vocal Dose: An Integrative Literature Review. *Speech, Language, Hearing Sciences and Education Journal* 19 (3) 429–438 https://doi.org/10.1590/1982-021620171932617

Baker, J., Barnett, C., Cavalli, L., Dietrich, M., Dixon, L., Duffy, J. R., Elias, A., Fraser, D. E., Freeburn, J. L., Gregory, C., McKenzie, K., Miller, N., Patterson, J., Roth, C., Roy, N., Short, J., Utianski, R., van Mersbergen, M., Vertigan, A., Carson, A., Stone, J. & McWhirter, L. (2021) Management of Functional Communication, Swallowing, Cough and Related Disorders: Consensus Recommendations for Speech and Language Therapy. *Journal of neurology, neurosurgery and psychiatry* 92 1112–1125 https://doi.org/10.1136/jnnp-2021-326767

Ballestas, S. A., Shelly, S., Soriano, R. M. & Klein, A. (2021) Trends in Recurrent Respiratory Papillomatosis Treatment. *Acta Otorrinolaringologica (English Edition)* 72 (2) 109–120 https://doi.org/10.1016/j.otoeng.2019.11.006

Bastian, R. W. & Thomas, J. P. (2016) Do Talkativeness and Vocal Loudness Correlate With Laryngeal Pathology? A Study of the Vocal Overdoer/Underdoer Continuum. *Journal of Voice* 30 (5) 557–562 https://doi.org/10.1016/j.jvoice.2015.06.012

Behlau, M., Madazio, G., Pacheco, C., Vaiano, T., Badaró, F. & Barbara, M. (in press) Coaching Strategies for Behavioural Voice Therapy and Training. *Journal of Voice* https://doi.org/10.1016/j.jvoice.2020.12.039

Belafsky, M.A., Shelly. S., Rothenberger, S. D., Ziegler, A., Hoffman, B., Hapner, E. R., Gartner-Schmidt, J. L, & Gillespie, A. I. (in press) Phonation Resistance Training Exercises (PhoRTE) With and Without Expiratory Muscle Strength Training (EMST) For Patients With Presbyphonia: A Noninferiority Randomized Clinical

Trial. *Journal of Voice* https://doi.org/10.1016/j.jvoice.2021.02.015

de Almeida, R. B. S., Costa, C. C., Lamounier e Silva Duarte, P., Rocha, A. K. P. B., Bernardes, M. N. D., Garcia, J. L., Freitas, L. B. & Ramos, H. V. L. (in press) Surgical Treatment Applied to Bilateral Vocal Fold Paralysis in Adults: Systematic Review. *Journal of Voice* https://doi.org/10.1016/j.jvoice.2020.11.018

Dehqan, A. & Scherer, R. C. (2019) Positive Effects of Manual Circumlaryngeal Therapy in the Treatment of Muscle Tension Dysphonia (MTD): Long Term Treatment Outcomes. *Journal of Voice* 33 (6) 866–871 https://doi.org/10.1016/j.jvoice.2018.07.010

Desjardins, M., Halstead, L., Simpson, A., Flume, P. & Bonilha, H. S. (2022) The Impact of Respiratory Function on Voice in Patients with Presbyphonia. *Journal of Voice* 36 (2) 256–271 https://doi.org/10.1016/j.jvoice.2020.05.027

Desjardins, M., Halstead, L., Simpson, A., Flume, P. & Bonilha, H. S. (2022) Respiratory Muscle Strength Training To Improve Vocal Function in Patients with Presbyphonia. *Journal of Voice* 36 (3) 344–360 https://doi.org/10.1016/j.jvoice.2020.06.006

Ebersole, B., Soni, R. S., Moran, K., Lango, M., Devarajan, K. & Jamal, N. (2017) The Influence of Occupation on Self-perceived Vocal Problems in Patients With Voice Complaints. *Journal of Voice* 32 (6) 673–680 https://doi.org/10.1016/j.jvoice.2017.08.028

Faham, M., Ahmadi, A., Silverman, E., Harouni, G.G. & Dabirmoghaddam, P. (2021) Quality of Life After Botulinum Toxin Injection in Patients with Adductor Spasmodic Dysphonia: a Systematic Review and Meta-Analysis. *Journal of Voice* 35 (2) 271–283 https://doi.org/10.1016/j.jvoice.2019.07.025

Gillespie, A. I. & Verdolini Abbott, K. (2011) The Influence of Clinical Terminology on Self-Efficacy for Voice. *Logopedics Phoniatrics Vocology* 36 (3) 91–99 https://doi.org/10.3109/14015439.2010.539259

Gray, H., Coman, L., Walton, C., Thorning, S., Cardell, E. & Weir, K. A. (in press) A Comparison of Voice and Psychotherapeutic Treatments For Adults With Functional Voice Disorders: A Systematic Review. *Journal of Voice* https://doi.org/10.1016/j.jvoice.2021.09.018

Hacki, T., Moerman, M. & Rubin. J. S. (2022) 'Malregulative' Rather Than 'Functional' Dysphonia: A New Etiological Terminology Framework for Phonation Disorders – A Position Paper by the Union of European Phoniatricians (UEP). *Journal of Voice 36* (1) 50–53 https://doi.org/10.1016/j.jvoice.2020.04.032

Halvorsen, T., Schwartz Walsted, E., Bucca, C., Bush, A., Cantarella, G., Friedrich, G., Herth, F. J. F., hull, J. H., Jung, H., Maat, R., Nordang, L., Remacle, M., Rasmussen, N., Wilson, J. A. & Heimdal, J-H. (2017) Inducible Laryngeal Obstruction: An Official Joint European Respiratory Society and European Laryngological Society Statement. *European Respiratory Journal 50* (3) https://doi.org/10.1183/13993003.02221-2016

Hintze, J. M., Ludlow, C. L., Bansberg, S. F., Adler, C. H. & Lott, D. G. (2017) Spasmodic Dysphonia: A Review. Part 1: Pathogenic Factors. *Otolaryngology-Head and Neck Surgery 157* (4) 551–557 https://doi.org/10.1177/0194599817728521

Hutchins, S. D. (2018) Singing in the Session. *The ASHA Leader 23* (6) https://doi.org/10.1044/leader.LML.23062018.26

Joshi, A. & Johns, M. M. (2018) Current Practices for Voice Rest Recommendations After Phonosurgery. *The Laryngoscope 128* 1170–1175 10.1002/lary.26979

Jo, Y. S., Kim, M. Y. & So, Y. K. (2021) Impact of Remnant Nodules on Immediate and Long-term Outcomes of Voice Therapy for Vocal Fold Nodules. *Journal of Voice 35* (3) 400–405 https://doi.org/10.1016/j.jvoice.2019.10.001

Kaneko, M., Shiromoto, O., Fujiu-Kurachi, M., Kishimoto, Y., Tateya, I. & Hirano, S. (2017) Optimal Duration for Voice

Rest After Vocal Fold Surgery: Randomized Controlled Clinical Study. *Journal of Voice 31* (1) 97–103 https://doi.org/10.1016/j.jvoice.2016.02.009

Kang, C. H., Zhang, N. & Lott, D. G. (2021) Muscle Tension Dysphagia: Contributing Factors and Treatment Efficacy. *Annals of Otology, Rhinology & Laryngology 130* (7) 674–681 https://doi.org/10.1177/0003489420966339

Khodeir, M. S., Hassan, S. M., El Shoubary, A. M. & Saad, M. N. A. (2021) Surgical and Nonsurgical Lines of Treatment of Reinke's Edema: A Systematic Literature Review. *Journal of Voice 35* (3) 502.e1–502.e11 https://doi.org/10.1016/j.jvoice.2019.10.016

Lee, Y. S., Lee, D. H., Jeong, G-E., Kim, J. W., Roh, J-L., Choi, S-H., Kim, S. Y. & Nam, S. Y. (2017) Treatment Efficacy of Voice Therapy for Vocal Fold Polyps and Factors Predictive of Its Efficacy. *Journal of Voice 31* (1) 120.e9–120.e13 https://doi.org/10.1016/j.jvoice.2016.02.014

Leeuw, M., Goossens, M. E. J. B., Linton, S. J., Crombez, G., Boersma, K. & Vlaeyen, J. W. S. (2007) The Fear-Avoidance Model of Musculoskeletal Pain: Current State of Scientific Evidence. *Journal of Behavioral Medicine 30* (1) 77–94 https://doi.org/10.1007/s10865-006-9085-0

Madill, C., Chacom, A., Kirby, E., Novakovic, D. & Nguyen, D. D. (2021) Active Ingredients of Voice Therapy for Muscle Tension Voice Disorders: A Retrospective Data Audit. *Journal of Clinical Medicine 10* (18) 4135 https://doi.org/10.3390/jcm10184135

Martins, R. H. G., Tavaress, E. L. M. & Pessin, A. B. P. (2017) Are Vocal Alterations Caused by Smoking in Reinke's Edema in Women Entirely Reversible After Microsurgery and Smoking Cessation? *Journal of Voice 31* (3) 380.e11–380.e14 https://doi.org/10.1016/j.jvoice.2016.06.012

Meyer, T. K., Spiekerman, C., Kaye, R., Blitzer, A., Kamizi, R. S., Jiang, L., & Weaver, E. M. (2021) Association of Laryngeal Botulinum Neurotoxin Injection with Work Productivity For Patients With Spasmodic Dysphonia. *JAMA Otolaryngology-Head and Neck Surgery 147* (9) 804–810 https://doi.org/10.1001/jamaoto.2021.1745

Nakagawa, H., Miyamoto, M., Kusuyama, T., Mori, Y., and Fukuda, H. (2012) Resolution of Vocal Fold Polyps With Conservative Treatment. *Journal of Voice 26* (3) e107-e110 https://doi.org/10.1016/j.jvoice.2011.07.005

Öcal, B., Tatar, E. Ç., Toptaş, G., Barmak, E., Saylam, G. & Korkmaz, M. H. (2020) Evaluation of Voice Quality in Patients With Vocal Fold Polyps: The Size of a Polyp Matters or Does It? *Journal of Voice 34* (2) 294–299 https://doi.org/10.1016/j.voice.2019.04.009

Park, J. H., Chae, M., An Y-H., Shim, H. J. & Kwon, M. (in press) Coprevalence of Presbycusis and Its Effect on Outcome of Voice Therapy in Patients with Presbyphonia. *Journal of Voice* https://doi.org/10.1016/j.jvoice.2020.09.030

Parker, L. A., Kunduk, M., Blouin, D. Adkins, L. & McWhorter, A. J. (2020) Voice Outcomes Following Multiple Surgeries for Recurrent Respiratory Papillomatosis. *Journal of Voice 34* (5) 791–798 https://doi.org/10.1016/j.voice.2019.02.004

Rihkanen, H. & Geneid, A. (2019) Voice Rest and Sick Leave after Phonosurgical Procedures: Surveys among European Laryngologists and Phoniatricians. *European Archives of Oto-Rhino-Laryngology 276* 483–487 https://doi.org/10.1007/s00405-019-05283-1

Shembel, A. C., Rosen, C. A., Zullo, T. G. & Gartner-Schmidt, J. L. (2013) Development and Validation of the Cough Severity Index: A Severity Index for Chronic Cough Related to the Upper Airway. *The Laryngoscope 123* (8)1931–1936 https://doi.org/10.1002/lary.23916

Shewell, C. (2009) *Voice Work. Art and Science in Changing Voices*. Chichester: Wiley-Blackwell

Stachler, R. J., Francis, D. O., Schwartz, S. R., Damask, C. C., Digoy, G. P., Krouse, H. J., McCoy, S. J., Ouellette, D. R., Patel, R. R., Reavis, C. W., Smith, L. J., Smith, M., Strode, S. W., Woo, P. & Nnacheta, L. C. (2018) Clinical Practice Guideline: Hoarseness (Dysphonia) (Update). *Otolaryngology-Head and Neck Surgery (158)* (1_suppl) S1-S42 https://doi.org/10.1177/0194599817751030

Sundar, K. M., Stark, A. C. & Hu, N. (2021) Is Laryngeal Hypersensitivity the Basis of Unexplained or Refractory Chronic Cough? *ERJ Open Research 7* (1) https://doi.org/10.1183/23120541.00793-2020

Tezcaner, Z. Ç., Gökmen, M. F. & Dursun, G. (2019) Clinical Features of Psychogenic Voice Disorders and the Efficiency of Voice Therapy and Psychological Evaluation. *Journal of Voice 33* (2) 250–254 https://doi.org/10.1016/j.jvoice.2017.09.022

Vanderaa, V. & Vinney, L. A. (in press) Laryngeal Sensory Symptoms in Spasmodic Dysphonia. *Journal of Voice* https://doi.org/10.1016/j.jvoice.2020.12.047

White, A. C., Awad, R. & Carding, P. (in press) Pre and Postoperative Voice Therapy Intervention for Benign Vocal Fold Lesions: A Systematic Review. *Journal of Voice.* https://doi.org/10.1016/j.jvoice.2021.06.005

White, A. C. & Carding, P. (2020) Pre-and Postoperative Voice Therapy for Benign Vocal Fold Lesions: Factors Influencing a Complex Intervention. *Journal of Voice 36* (1) 59–67 https://doi.org/10.1016/j.jvoice.2020.04.004

Yorkston, K., Baylor, C. R., Eadie, T. & Kapsner-Smith, M. (2021) Perceptions Regarding Communicative Participation in Individuals Receiving Botulinum Toxin Injections for Laryngeal Dystonia. *International Journal of Language & Communication Disorders 56* (6) 1296–1315 https://doi.org/10.1111/1460-6984.13668

Young, V. N. (2020) Patients' Attitudes Regarding Treatment for Vocal Fold Atrophy. *Journal of Voice 34* (5) 763–768 https://doi.org/10.1016/j.jvoice.2019.04.012

Zhuge, P., You, H., Wang, H., Zhang, Y. & Du, H. (2016) An Analysis of the Effects of Voice Therapy on Patients With Early Vocal Fold Polyps. *Journal of Voice 30* (6) 698–701 https://doi.org/10.1016/j.jvoice.2015.08.013

Ziegler, A. & Hapner, E. R. (2020) Vocal Dose in Older Adults with Presbyphonia: An Analytic, Cross-Sectional Study. *Journal of Voice 34* (2) 221–230 https://doi.org/10.1016/j.jvoice.2018.09.005

ADDITIONAL LEARNING RESOURCES

RCSLT factsheet for people with upper airway disorders www.rcslt.org/wp-content/uploads/media/Project/RCSLT/rcslt-upper-airway-disorders-factsheet.pdf

British Voice Association factsheet for people with vocal fold palsies www.britishvoiceassociation.org.uk/downloads/free-voice-care-literature/Paralysed%20Vocal%20Folds%20and%20Voice.pdf

Chapter 7

WORKING WITH PROFESSIONAL VOICE USERS

As you gain experience and work with a range of clients, you will soon notice a frequency of referrals associated with specific groups of voice users who have high levels of occupational vocal demand. With patterns of vocal hazards across and within professions, the unique risk factors associated with each group can be addressed through therapy tailored to the client's profession, as well as the individual. The four specific groups of vocal athletes considered in this chapter include: educators; contact centre employees; those working in the sports and fitness industry; and performers. We will also consider the relevance of vocal warm-ups and cool-downs and preventative intervention for professional voice users.

TIP 40 – VOCAL ATHLETES

Shewell (2009) identifies six voice user groups with high voice demands: supporters; callers; transmitters; informers; leaders and sellers; and performers. Some of these groups will operate at a non-professional level, some will be semi-professional, and others will be professional or elite-level vocal athletes. Note that the term "professional" is commonly used to describe voice users who rely on their voices as a key occupational tool, but is also used to delineate level of expertise within communicative function.

Regardless of the performance level, all voice user groups in this chapter are vocal athletes and I encourage you to share this term with your clients. Being reliant on their voices, professional voice users may be more attuned to the subtle differences in their voice quality and function, odynophonia (pain on speaking), and increased vocal effort and fatigue (Ebersole et al., 2017). This awareness can contribute to a search for early intervention which optimises treatment outcomes, though you will also meet many professional voice users who have yet to recognise the voice as the tool of their trade and the higher level of care and attention required.

Some clients ask why they experience voice difficulties when their colleagues do not. This is likely to be due to a combination of personal factors, an individual vocal demand response (Tip 15) and vocal vulnerabilities being revealed through high levels of vocal demand. Had your client chosen a less vocally demanding career path, some of the difficulties may have gone unnoticed, so although our intervention doesn't necessarily change the client's personal susceptibility to voice difficulties it will support them to manage the risks and optimise individual function.

The rest of this chapter considers the most common professional voice user groups seen in clinic but, from clinical experience, it is also worth briefly mentioning the vocal risks for taxi drivers, airline staff, tour guides and, importantly, health professionals. As reiterated in Tips 41, 42, 43, and 44, use your curiosity about your clients' work practices and environment to gather comprehensive data which allow you to identify the occupational risks.

Taxi drivers

In any usual face-to-face conversation, the voice travels from the speaker to the listener in a straight line but when a taxi driver is speaking, their voice often needs to do a U-turn to reach the passengers' ears in the back of the cab. Turning the neck round to help the driver's voice travel and as an attempt to connect with the passenger(s) in the rear view mirror contributes to a mis-aligned upper body position, adding tension and strain around the neck and larynx. Sitting in one position for prolonged periods is similarly poor for posture and the voice.

Airline industry workers

Although take-off and landing offer some reprieve from speaking, cabin crew are reliant on their voices to convey important safety information, to enquire about passenger comfort, and to promote on-board services. The cabin environment can be drying, and projecting the voice along the length of an aircraft above engine noise and passenger conversation can increase the risk of strain. Air traffic controllers have been recognised as potentially being vulnerable to voice difficulties, influenced by their high-pressure working environment (Villar et al., 2016; Korn et al., 2019) and from clinical experience, this can be true for pilots too.

Tour guides

Sanssené et al.'s (2020) research suggests tour guides are at higher risk of voice difficulties than the general population, and certainly commentaries provided on an open-top bus, in a busy museum with background noise, on an open-air walking tour with changeable weather conditions, or in buildings with high ceilings and wide spaces are all susceptible to acoustic challenges. Microphones are not suitable for all environments and in quiet places, such as an art gallery, a tour guide may face the opposite challenge of trying to contain a voice so as not to be heard.

Health professionals

Of course, any health professional relies on their voice to ask questions and convey instructions to clients and the occupational vocal hazards identified for SLTs and SLT students in Tip 2 are relevant for other health professionals too. Hard-of-hearing clients demand greater vocal intensity, crouching down at a hospital bedside or working with children on the floor alters posture, and busy caseloads can increase stress.

Preventative education

Preventative voice care education is often proposed as a means of reducing professional voice users' risk of developing dysphonia, and the call for this has been made for fitness instructors and gym managers (Rumbach, 2013; Aiken & Rumbach, 2018; Estes et al., 2020), student teachers (Alves et al., 2021; Greve et al., 2019; Meier & Beushausen, 2021), and teachers (Van Houtte et al., 2011). It can be particularly important where speakers are not aware of the need to look after their voices (Grillo & Brosious, 2019), and dedicated education may increase willingness to implement vocal care advice (Porcaro et al., 2021) and nurture healthier responses to symptoms of a difficult voice (Pomaville et al., 2020) with improved retention of information from repeated education (Aiken & Rumbach, 2018; Flynn, 2020). However, any programme dedicated to an individual client group must reflect the vocal demands and specific challenges associated with that group (Zenari et al., in press). There may be overlap in how you explain voice care for educators and fitness instructors, for example, but you should also highlight the specific risks associated with the different professions. You should also consider whether you will provide in-person education, online instruction, or make use of apps (Aiken & Rumbach, 2018).

TIP 41 – EDUCATORS

We know teachers are at greater risk of dysphonia than the normal population (Van Houtte et al., 2011) due to a combination of background noise, singing, increased vocal intensity, and large prosodic variations (Assad et al., 2017), and a stressful working environment with possible burnout (de Brito Mota et al., 2019). Such risk factors reiterate the importance of approaching the voice holistically and many of my teaching clients have expressed gratitude for the opportunity to invest in their long-term career, spreading vocal care advice to their colleagues. Individual clients may be interested in purchasing *The Voice in Education* by Martin and Darnley (2019) as an accessible resource to support their ongoing voice care and development, or they could recommend this to their headteacher as an investment in their whole staff group. It is also a very comprehensive resource for SLTs.

Some of the guidance in this tip is common to all clients working in education and some of it is more relevant for specific education settings. Let's take a look at the common aspects of an educational voice you will need to consider.

Teaching environment

Teaching rooms usually require educators to project their voices more loudly and over greater distances than in normal conversation. Background noise levels are influenced by the age of the pupils, the number of students in the class, and the subject being taught, so the noise generated by young children playing excitedly with Lego ® may match those of secondary school children cooking with pots and pans or university students working in an engineering laboratory. Additional competing noise may also come from seemingly innocuous sources – one of my teaching clients had a hand-dryer on the other side of their classroom wall which necessitated greater vocal intensity each time it was used!

Teaching demands

Primary education workers usually have a consistent age of pupils across the academic year, but may change age group at the start of each year. As younger children usually require greater support than older children, early years educators often report higher vocal demand than those in the later years of primary or elementary school. Going by the same principle, elementary or primary educators may, in turn, report less vocal demand than secondary or high school educators unless the subject relies on verbal interaction such as modern languages, drama, music, sports, or modern studies.

In secondary education, where teaching is subject-specific rather than age-specific, your clients may have different teaching demands on different days depending on the learning needs of their pupils and their timetable. There may also be seasonal variation in voice demands – PE teachers working outdoors, for instance, may find it more difficult to project their voice above the wind and rain in the colder months, and music teachers may find it more difficult at the end of each term if there are rehearsals and performances to prepare for.

Teaching style

Just as we all have our own individual therapeutic style, educators have their own style of teaching. Clients with a naturally quiet voice may struggle to be heard against noise, and others who are comfortable using a strong, resonant voice in the classroom may struggle to contain this for smaller spaces such as staff rooms or tutorials.

Particularly for educators working with younger pupils, an excessively high-pitched voice conveying enthusiasm elevates the larynx, which becomes tiring if this position is held for long periods. The fatigue is further compounded by teachers attempting to use character voices during storytelling or reading time as moving between very different pitches is difficult without a flexible larynx. An elevated larynx may lend itself to a witch's voice, for example, but is far from the deep pitch of Daddy Bear in the story of Goldilocks, and in secondary education a drama teacher attempting to move between sombre tones befitting Shakespeare with one class and a lighter female voice in West Side Story may also find pitch variation challenging. Your role will be to educate your clients about the challenges of moving between extremes of pitches and show how enthusiasm can be conveyed effectively and safely through language, pausing, and non-verbal communication.

Teaching support

Additional staff are usually reserved for classes with children with additional support needs or where practical support is needed for experiments and construction activities, but it may be prudent for your client to request teaching support if they are struggling to manage voice demands single-handedly. Temporary support allows vocal healing while you and your client work to develop a more robust voice for the future or longer term cover provides support for particularly vocally demanding activities. The benefits of additional staff include:

- sharing the provision of whole-class instructions.
- sharing the responsibility for the classroom so each educator ensures their allocated pupils pay attention, listen, or complete a task. This means neither educator has to project their voice across the whole room.
- looking after the class while each other nips to the bathroom because they've been staying well hydrated. Some teachers are reluctant to increase their fluid intake if going to the bathroom between dedicated break times leaves their pupils unsupervised.

Reducing vocal load can be further achieved by:

- using alternatives to the voice to attract attention. This could be a silent signal such as raising a hand, or a whistle to cut across classroom noise and reach further distances outside. Note that some pupils are sensitive to loud noises

due to health diagnoses or family circumstances so do check this would work for your client's students.
- requesting a roaming microphone with portable speaker to reduce the vocal intensity required. These may be funded by school funds or through Access to Work (Tip 49). Microphones are more likely to be available in tertiary education lecture theatres but if these are fixed to a computer stand or lectern at the front of the class, not only do they prevent the educator from moving around with a free body, their height may not be suitable for all teaching staff, which in turn alters posture and creates bodily tension.

Improving vocal health

Reducing tension and warming up the voice

Voiceless, portable tension-reducing exercises, such as lip trills and yawning (Tip 26) can be practised during a commute, and more extensive warm-ups (Tip 45) can be completed at the place of work before students and colleagues arrive. They can even be done behind a toilet door if your client does not have access to private space!

Posture

Crouching next to children or sitting on low chairs hinders easy breathing in compressing the respiratory system and contributes to bodily tension radiating into the voice. Head, neck, and body stretches can contribute to tension relief and pupils could be encouraged to join in, either as part of fun movement for younger children or with explicit discussion about body well-being for older students.

Using the breath more effectively

Tip 25 highlighted the consequences of running out of air if speakers do not pause for breath, and familiar utterances said with automaticity can increase this risk. Just as I have therapeutic statements or instructions which I say regularly, educators may have well-rehearsed statements around preparing their class for the time ahead or instructions for particular tasks. This sentence is an example of such a phrase, even though the specific content would vary from class to class, day to day, or from educator to educator.

> *"so, this morning we're going to practise our eight times table then we'll have story time and just before lunch you'll be with Miss Blair for PE".*

Although it may be possible to say all 33 syllables on one breath, doing so risks laryngeal strain and reinforces a pattern of breathing which is not conducive to safe voice use. Breaking this down to clauses with identified breath groups as in Tip 25 ensures better breath support and develops client awareness of the respiratory difference between long, unsupported utterances and long, fully supported utterances. My suggested breath groups are below but these are based on my communication and physiology, and I'm also imagining providing this information in a way that young children can follow so am being particularly careful about breaking up the clauses. You will need to identify what works for your client for the utterances they bring to practice.

> *"so* (1 syllable) - *this morning we're going to practise* (9 syllables) - *our eight times table* (5 syllables) - *then we'll have story time* (6 syllables) - *and just before lunch* (5 syllables) - *you'll be with Miss Blair for PE* (8 syllables)*".*

Projection of the voice

In addition to pausing for more regular replenishment of the breath, improved breath support contributes to stronger projection rather than relying on laryngeal strain, and this can be supplemented with mild twang quality to cut through loud noise.

Temporary leave from teaching

Although sharing vocal load with a colleague offers some voice rest for your client, an educator with a diagnosis of vocal fold nodules, or other pathology which requires time to heal, may need a period of no direct teaching. Swapping pupil contact for desk duties allows them to remain at work but, if they are likely to be asked to cover classes or find it hard to resist talking in the company of others, a period of sick leave should be considered. This sick leave will not be authorised by you as it requires GP or physician approval and, as with many healthcare professionals, teachers often find it difficult to request sick leave in relation to their voice. Not looking physically unwell can lead to colleague assumption that they are still fit for work, despite audible hoarseness indicating otherwise. Educators also report that returning to work after any leave can be challenging, particularly if they need to revise their teaching plans and so they plough on to avoid this. They are invariably passionate about their job with dedication to student learning but occupational commitment can become our clients' downfall when loyalty to their job is at the expense of self-care. We need to show them that they can be great educators *and* have a great voice.

TIP 42 – CONTACT CENTRE WORKERS

Contact centre workers include those working in telephone banking, TV and internet contracts, and handling emergency calls. Shifts vary from four to ten hours, with different company rules around breaks and widely varying expectations around the number of calls being managed by individual employees. Your case history gathering therefore needs to include questions about the type of work (e.g. frontline call handling compared with managerial services or technical services), the shift pattern, the equipment used, specific information to be provided during calls, and your client's relationship with their work.

Shift patterns

Employees are entitled to a statutory number of breaks in accordance with shift length. At the time of publication, UK workers are entitled to one, uninterrupted 20-minute break when working for longer than six hours, and additional breaks will depend on the employer. For clients with difficulties exacerbated by long periods of speaking it may be more helpful to split their breaks for greater frequency of voice rest. Although this may not be standard practice, employers do have an occupational health responsibility and should be providing reasonable adjustments if required.

It is impossible to define safe occupational voice limits since a numerical value of hours' use or decibels of intensity doesn't take into account interpersonal differences in the voice, or other influencing factors such as stress, environmental conditions, or general health status (Cantarella et al., 2014). Your recommendations regarding shift patterns will therefore need to be contextualised to your individual client's situation and health history.

Equipment

All contact centre workers should use a supportive chair to facilitate an upright posture, and a headset with microphone.

Double earpieces block out surrounding noise better than single earpieces, and as distracting background noise can lead to upper body tension from straining to hear the customer, we need to check our clients are not altering their head and neck position in response to their work environment.

If a client reports poor availability of equipment or difficulties with a single earpiece headset you should suggest they approach their Human Resources department to request additional and/or alternative equipment.

Responding to calls

Unlike educators whose regular phrases are self-generated, there are often standard company scripts for answering the phone or explaining the terms and conditions of a contract. New employees will rely on this script which facilitates identification of the appropriate breath groups, but as the script becomes increasingly familiar, there is growing risk of sentences running into each other to create one long sentence on a single allocated breath. The more frequently the client does not pause for breath, the more they adopt this approach, which can gradually extend to non-work situations, further reinforcing this maladaptive habit.

As with educators, follow the guidance in Tip 25 to support your client in developing effective breath support, using the statements your client uses to make this relevant for the workplace. For example:

> *Hello* (2 syllables) - *Voice Navigation, Editing Department* (11 syllables) - *Carolyn speaking* (5 syllables) - *how can I help you* (5 syllables)?

You can also try this with your clients' statements around terms and conditions or standard questions to give them an opportunity to identify the breath groups independently, remembering that increasing cognitive effort (Tip 9) facilitates client progress.

A sense of urgency in conversation due to company pressure to answer a certain number of calls or the time-critical nature of emergency call conversations may challenge your client to develop more effective use of the breath and you can offer reassurance that the fractions of seconds needed for the additional breaths are far outweighed by the benefit of full breath support and decreased risk of laryngeal strain.

Relationship with work

Pressure to answer calls promptly, and angry or upset customers make for a stressful working environment and this stress has a compounding impact on the voice (Tip 21) as well as the prolonged periods of speaking. Your tender conversation skills (Tip 7) will be important in validating the client's experience and supporting them to identify ways in which they can manage their stress.

TIP 43 – CLIENTS IN THE ARTS INDUSTRY

Sung or spoken performances range from an acoustic set in a quiet venue, a pub gig with competing noise from audience conversation, a cruise ship cabaret performance to 100 people, or a stadium gig with an audience of thousands. Regardless of location, where performing is a client's livelihood they need to have outstanding levels of vocal care and safe use. I also encourage you to read Chapter 29 (The acting voice) and Chapter 30 (The singing voice) in Shewell (2009) to develop your knowledge of working with performers in conjunction with the information below.

Evaluating the singing voice

You already know that alongside your acoustic-perceptual assessment, client self-perception is important (Tip 14). Although singers can have some broad voice complaints, generic self-rating scales may not capture the full experience for a singer (Renk et al., 2017). The Voice Handicap Index (VHI) (Jacobsen et al., 1997) and its shortened version, the Voice Handicap Index-10 (Rosen et al., 2004), have both been adapted for singers to produce the Singing Voice Handicap Index (SVHI) (Cohen et al., 2007) and the Singing Voice Handicap Index-10 (SVHI-10) (Cohen et al., 2009) which is in Appendix 1. Acoustic, perceptual, and self-rating outcome measurements may be supplemented by reports of increased stamina across a gig or series of gigs, and greater flexibility across the pitch range.

Can the show go on?

Performing through a known injury or existing pathology risks exacerbation of the problem and should be discouraged. However, despite clear warning signs that the voice is incapable of meeting performance demands, amateur and professional performers may experience internal and external pressures to continue their work. Where one client does not want to disappoint their Church choir at a Christmas concert, another performing in a major theatre in their own city may feel the pull of a home audience. Perceived audience expectations also contribute to performers continuing to work so the next time our favourite artist cancels a show, let's be forgiving! Elite performers with personal vocal coaches should be able to access support as soon as a problem arises, avoiding the need to wait for publicly funded therapy, and those in elite group shows may have a well-trained understudy for a temporary period of voice rest. Conversely, no paid sick leave and worry about future reputation can make it challenging for self-employed performers to take the rest but your skills in tender conversations (Tip 7) will allow you to firmly, but sensitively, inform your client of the vocal risks in continuing to perform whilst still also feeling heard by you. I have worked with clients who have heeded advice and also with those who have continued to perform despite advice to the contrary.

Testing whether a singing voice is capable of full rehearsal or performance can be done using the three steps of: *siren, miren, sing*. These are progressive steps in which sirening has the lowest vocal demand, the miren adds a layer of articulation to phonation, and the singing is the most challenging step of the three. As a systematic process, your client shouldn't progress to the next level until they have mastered the previous one(s). Try self-development activity 22 before explaining this to clients and to evaluate the effect on your voice.

Self-development activity 22 – sirening, mirening, and singing

Step 1 – sirening

Make an [ŋ], as in the end of "going", for 3 seconds so you can feel the contact between your tongue and velum. Now glide up and down the pitches on the [ŋ] sound. Singers will often use sirening as part of their warm-up routine and you should reiterate the value of this. Now, pick a song (for ease this could be something like happy birthday) and siren the song, that is, follow the melody on the [ŋ] without any other articulatory movement.

STEP 2 – MIRENING

The term mirening comes from a combination of mouthing and sirening so this time, when you siren your song, add in articulatory movement for an audible version of the words. The version will be nasalised since you're using [ŋ] and your articulation won't be as distinct as if singing normally but you're starting to evaluate the possibility of combining vocal flexibility and articulation.

- Can you reach the notes at either end of the range?
- Where do you start to have difficulty?

STEP 3 – SINGING

If sirening and mirening have been successful, now try singing the song, but if sirening and/or mirening are difficult to do, singing is going to be difficult. In fact, where singers report difficulty with specific songs, they shouldn't be singing them until they can master the sirening and mirening versions.

Performance warm-ups and cool-downs

I would expect elite performers to be fastidious about where, when, and how they warm up their voice pre-performance but performers at professional or semi-professional level may be at the mercy of external influences. These include non-private backstage facilities, traffic preventing an early arrival for full engagement with a vocal warm-up, or insufficient time being allocated for pre-performance preparation. Although many performers endeavour to complete vocal warm-ups, I've met far fewer singers who adopt a post-performance vocal care routine, even though these are the equivalent of the post-match stretches of an amateur or professional sportsperson.

Basic warm-up exercises and cool-downs are provided in Tip 45 for all professional voice users and these can be used as a starting point for singers without their own routine. They will need to supplement these with warm-up exercises tailored to their style of singing or performance and these can be developed with a vocal coach.

External support for performing clients

Many of our voice skills overlap with those of a vocal coach or singing teacher, and greater flexibility in the spoken voice developed in therapy can often enhance a client's flexibility in singing. However, specific singing guidance should be provided by a singing teacher or vocal coach unless you hold dual qualifications in singing and speech and language therapy. When encouraging a client to seek advice from a singing teacher, make sure they look for someone who has expertise in their genre of singing. There is little merit in a folk singer seeking advice from an opera singer! Even if the client's onward vocal growth will be nurtured by a singing professional, you can still provide general vocal health advice and if you are trained in manual therapy, this will be relevant for spoken and singing voices.

The British Association of Performing Arts Medicine (BAPAM) provides health and well-being services for clients working in the performing arts including support for vocal health, mental health, musculoskeletal health, and hearing issues. As well as workshops for performers and training for health professionals, their resources include a series of warm-up exercises which are applicable to both singing and non-singing musicians. A Fit to Sing factsheet has 12 tips on how to prepare for singing and the non-vocal aspects singers should consider such as overall health, the impact of excessive socialising, and the impact of their wider lifestyle on performance, and our client account by Amanda Lynne acknowledges the impact other activities had on her voice. I would recommend you become familiar with BAPAM resources so you are ready to share them if your client asks for advice regarding warm-ups.

TIP 44 – CLIENTS IN THE FITNESS INDUSTRY

As with other groups of professional voice users, our case history needs to gather specific data about our fitness clients' working patterns, environments, and voice use. The demands differ for yoga teachers and high-intensity indoor cycling instructors, for example, and will be different again if instruction is provided live and face-to-face, live but remotely, or asynchronously via pre-recorded instruction.

Some clients in the fitness industry are permanent employees in a commercial or private gym while others will be self-employed, either renting space in a private gym or peripatetically providing classes to several gyms. Regardless of contract type, the fitness industry may be a permanent career path for some workers while it is supplementary income for others, such as those in the creative industries without a regular salary or students looking for part-time work to pay tuition fees or rent.

Notable vocal challenges for clients in the fitness industry include: speaking during periods of increased cardiorespiratory effort; needing to use the voice creatively to motivate clients; projecting the voice against background noise; and environments with irritants such as air-conditioning or chlorinated water. We know the increased glottal closure from lifting something heavy helps with thoracic stability but this comes with compression of the vocal folds, and so breath holding during weight training can be irritating, with increased sensations of throat pain, changes in voice, or a globus sensation (Rumbach et al., 2020). Unfortunately, there may be inadequate provision of equipment to reduce vocal effort and poor education regarding occupational voice use (Aiken & Rumbach, 2018; Estes et al., 2020), and you may hear accounts of industry apathy around vocal health (Aiken & Rumbach, 2018).

In addition to direct voice therapy to address vocal technique problems, recommendations to consider with this client group are:

- Use a microphone so they can be heard from the front to the back of a gym space and over the whirr of equipment, loud motivating music, or other instructors. Our clients may be very fit but there is still a challenge combining speaking at high intensity and exertion.
- Ensure more frequent top-up breaths are taken to offset the increased respiratory effort from exercise.
- Avoid consecutive classes or lengthy instruction with high vocal demand, factoring in opportunity for rest during and between classes. Although amplification can reduce the physical effort for fitness instructors and allow them to say more in class (Allison et al., 2020) voice conservation is still advised.
- Use gestures and demonstration in lieu of verbal instruction.
- Rely on language to convey motivation rather than only tone of voice. Short phrases such as "good!", "that's it!", or "keep going!" can be as effective as longer utterances like "you're doing brilliantly – keep it up!" but reduce vocal demand. It may not seem much relief in these brief examples but extrapolating this across a full working day will soon add up.

TIP 45 – VOCAL WARM-UPS AND COOL-DOWNS

It is an SLT's responsibility to encourage vocal warm-ups and cool-downs with all professional voice users, and using the analogy of "vocal athletes" can be useful again here as reinforcement of your message. Just as a marathon runner ensures their muscles are well-warmed before a long period of activity, our vocal athletes should warm up the voice prior to long periods of speaking, and similarly just as an athlete would stretch after competition, clients should be cooling down their voices after use.

Pre-warm-up requirement

Before warming up the voice, the body and vocal tract need to be tension-free, as attempts to achieve a flexible voice will be fruitless if there is pre-existing tension. Indeed, a combination of a physical and a vocal warm-up can be more effective at facilitating a readiness to sing and keeping singers in tune than a physical or vocal warm-up alone (Cook-Cunningham & Grady, 2018). A client in the early stages of therapy may need to dedicate time to laryngeal deconstriction to reduce tension prior to warm-up exercises, but should be able to progress more quickly to warm-ups with continued practice.

Warm-ups

The BAPAM exercises in Tip 43 are applicable for all professional voice users and Martin and Darnley (2019) and Martin (2021) also contain very appropriate suggestions. Any warm-up routine should consider the articulators as well as the larynx, so lip trills, tongue twisters, and gurning are all beneficial alongside pitch variation.

Cool-downs

Immediate post-performance voice care should facilitate a transition from "performance mode" to "conversational mode". Singing style which alters position of the larynx can lead to fatigue and strain in the speaking voice if the larynx does not return to a more habitual position. A cool-down routine can include:

- downward pitch glides on lip trills to release tension and lower the larynx
- yawning on a downward pitch glide to lower the larynx
- glottal fry (creaky voice quality) to reduce vocal load
- head and neck stretches to counteract bodily tension used in anchoring
- continued hydration. If steam inhalations are used, post-inhalation voice rest can be incorporated into the drive home from a performance, but other clients will need to exercise caution if they intend to indulge in post-gig socialising with bandmates or performing colleagues.

REFERENCES

Aiken, P. J. & Rumbach, A. F. (2018) Keeping the Voice Fit in the Group Fitness Industry; A Qualitative Study to Determine What Instructors Want in a Voice Education Program. *Journal of Voice 32* (2) 256.e25–256.e34 https://doi.org/10.1016/j.jvoice.2017.04.014

Allison, L. H., Sandage, M. J., & Weaver, A. J. (2020) Vocal Dose for Rhythm-Based Indoor Cycling Instructors With and Without Amplification. *Journal of Voice 34* (6) 963.e23–963.e31 https://doi.org/10.1016/j.jvoice.2019.05.010

Alves, I. A. V., Paulino, V. C. P., Souza, A. L. R., Barbosa, M. A. & Porto, C. C. (2021) Voice Care from the Student Teachers' Perspective. *Journal of Voice 35* (4) 664.e21–664.e26 https://doi.org/10.1016/j.jvoice.2019.12.010

Assad, J. P., de castro Magalhães, Santos, J. N. & Gama, A. C. C. (2017) Vocal Dose: An Integrative Literature Review. *Speech, Language, Hearing Sciences and Education Journal 19* (3) 429–438 https://doi.org/10.1590/1982-021620171932617

Cantarella, , G., Iofrida, E., Boria, P., Giordana, S., Binatti, O., Pignatoro, L., Manfredim C., Forti, S. & Dejonckere, P. (2014) Ambulatory Phonation Monitoring in a Sample of 92 Call Center Operators. *Journal of Voice 28* (3) 393.e1–393.e6 https://doi.org/10.1016/j.jvoice.2013.10.002

Cohen, S. M., Jacobson, B., Garrett, C. G. & Noordzij, J. P. (2007) Creation and Validation of the Singing Voice Handicap Index. *The Annals of Otology, Rhinology and Laryngology 116* (6) 402–406 https://doi.org/10.1177/000348940711600602

Cohen, S. M., Statham, M., Rosen, C. A. & Zullo, T. (2009) Development and Validation of the Singing Voice Handicap-10. *The Laryngoscope 119* (9) 1864–1869 https://doi.org/10.1002/lary.20580

Cook-Cunningham, S. L. & Grady, M. L. (2018) The Effects of Three Physical and Vocal Warm-Up Procedures on Acoustic and Perceptual Measures of Choral Sound. *Journal of Voice 32* 2 192–199 https://doi.org/10.1016/j.jvoice.2017.04.003

de Brito Mota, A. F., Giannini, S. P. P., de Oliviera, I. B., Paparelli, R., Dornelas, R. & Ferreira, L. P. (2019) Voice Disorder and Burnout Syndrome in Teachers. *Journal of Voice 33* (4) https://doi.org/10.1016/j.jvoice.2018.01.022

Ebersole, B., Soni, R. S., Moran, K., Lango, M., Devarajan, K. & Jamal, N. (2017) The Influence of Occupation on Self-perceived Vocal Problems in Patients With Voice Complaints. *Journal of Voice 32* (6) 673–680 https://doi.org/10.1016/j.jvoice.2017.08.028

Estes, C., Sadaoughi, B., Coleman, R., D'Angelo, D. & Sulica, L. (2020) Phonotraumatic Injury in Fitness Instructors: Risk Factors, Diagnoses and Treatment Methods. *Journal of Voice 34* (2) 272–279 https://doi.org/10.1016/j.jvoice.2018.10.001

Flynn, A. (2020) Vocal Health Education in Undergraduate Performing Arts Training Programs. *Journal of Voice 34* (5) 806.e33–806.e44 https://doi.org/10.1016/j.jvoice.2019.03.016

Greve, K., Bryn, E. K. & Simberg, S. (2019) Voice Disorders and Impact of Voice Handicap in Norwegian Student Teachers. *Journal of Voice 33* (4) 445–452 https://doi.org/10.1016/j.jvoice.2018.01.019

Grillo, E. U. & Brosious, J. N. (2019) Results of a Voice-Related Survey of Physical Education Student Teachers. *Communication Disorders Quarterly 40* (2) 99–108 https://doi.org/10.1177/1525740118774207

Jacobsen, B. H., Johnson, A., Grywalski, C., Silbergleit, A., Jacobsen, G. (1997) The Voice Handicap Index (VHI) Development and Validation. *American Journal of Speech-Language Pathology 6* (3) 66–70 https://doi.org/10.1044/1058-0360.0603.66

Korn, G. P., Villar, A. C. & Azevedo, R. R. (2019) Hoarseness and Vocal Tract Discomfort and Associated Risk Factors in Air Traffic Controllers. *Brazilian Journal of Otorhinolaryngology 85* (3) 329–336 https://doi.org/10.1016/j.bjorl.2018.02.009

Martin, S. (2021) *Working With Voice Disorders. Theory and Practice.* (3rd Ed.) Abingdon: Routledge.

Martin, S. & Darnley, L. (2019) *The Voice in Education.* Oxford: Compton Publishing.

Meier, B. & Beushausen, U. (2021) Long-Term Effects of a Voice Training Program to Prevent Voice Disorders in Teachers. *Journal of Voice 35* (2) 324.e1–324.e8 https://doi.org/10.1016/j.jvoice.2019.06.003

Pomaville, F., Tekerlek, K. & Radford, A. (2020) The Effectiveness of Vocal Hygiene Education for Decreasing At-Risk Vocal Behaviors in Vocal Performers. *The Journal of Voice 34* (5) 709–719 https://doi.org/10.1016j.jvoice.2019.03.004

Porcaro, C. K., Howery, S., Suhanddron, A. & Gollery, T. (2021) Impact of Vocal Hygiene Training on Teachers' Willingness to Change Vocal Behaviours. *Journal of Voice 35* (3) 499.e1–499.e11 https://doi.org/10.1016/j.jvoice.2019.11.011

Renk, E., Sulica, L., Grossman, C., Georges, J. & Murry, T. (2017) VHI-10 and SVHI-10 Differences in Singers' Self-perception of Dysphonia Severity. *Journal of Voice*

31 (3) 383.e1–383.e4 https://doi.org/10.1016/j.jvoice.2016.08.017

Rosen, C. A., Lee, A. S., Osborne, J., Zullo, T. & Murry, T. (2004) Development and validation of the voice handicap index-10. *Laryngoscope 114* 9 1549–1556 https://doi.org/10.1097/00005537-200409000-00009

Rumbach, A. F. (2013) Vocal Problems of Group Fitness Instructors: Prevalence of Self-Reported Sensory and Auditory-Perceptual Voice Symptoms and the Need for Preventative Education and Training. *Journal of Voice 27* (4) 524.e11–524.e21 https://doi.org/10.1016/j.jvoice.2013.01.016

Rumbach, A. F., Maddox, M., Hull, M. & Khidr, A. (2020) Laryngeal Symptoms in Weightlifting Athletes. *Journal of Voice 34* (6) 964.e1–964.e10 https://doi.org/10.1016/j.j.voice.2019.06.004

Sanssené, C., Bardi, J. & Welby-Gieusse, M. (2020) Prevalence and Risk Factors of Voice Disorders in French Tour Guides. *Journal of Voice 34* (6) 911–917 https://doi.org/10.1016/j.jvoice.2019.05.002

Shewell, C. (2009) *Voice Work. Art and Science in Changing Voices.* Chichester: Wiley-Blackwell.

Van Houtte, E., Claeys, S., Wuyts, F. & Van Lierde, K. (2011) The Impact of Voice Disorders Among Teachers: Vocal Complaints, Treatment-Seeking Behaviour, Knowledge of Vocal Care, and Voice-Related Absenteeism. *Journal of Voice 25* (5) 570–575 https://doi.org/10.1016/j.jvoice.2010.04.008

Villar, A. C. N. W. B., Korn, G. P. & Azevedo, R. R. (2016) Perceptual-auditory and Acoustic Analysis of Air Traffic Controllers' Voices Pre- and Postshift. *Journal of Voice 30* (6) 768.e11–768.e15 https://doi.org/10.1016/j.jvoice.2015.10.021

Zenari, M. S., dos Reis Cota, A. de Albuquerque Rodrigues, D. & Nemr, K. (in press) Do Professionals Who Use the Voice in a Journalistic Context Benefit from Humming as a Semi-occluded Vocal Tract Exercise? *Journal of Voice* https://doi.org/10.1016/j.jvoice.2021.03.011

ADDITIONAL LEARNING RESOURCES

British Association of Performing Arts Medicine – Warm-up Exercises for Musicians www.bapam.org.uk/wp-content/uploads/2020/05/BAPAM-Factsheet-Warm-Ups-Dont-Cramp-Your-Style-2020.pdf

British Association of Performing Arts Medicine – Fit to Sing Factsheet www.bapam.org.uk/wp-content/uploads/2020/05/Fit-to-Sing-BAPAM-Factsheet-2020.pdf

Chapter 8

PROFESSIONAL LIAISON

One of the really enjoyable elements of SLT work, in any specialism, is multi-disciplinary working. Not only do we broaden our knowledge through learning from others but liaison with colleagues in other professions fosters a sense of community as we work towards positive outcomes and healthy well-being for our clients. Working in the field of voice is no different and in this chapter you will learn about the healthcare professionals responsible for our clients' physical health, mental health, smoking cessation, and employment. Three hypothetical client examples are provided to start you thinking about how this might work in reality.

TIP 46 – SUPPORT FOR ... PHYSICAL HEALTH
Ear, Nose and Throat consultants

Endoscopic evaluation of the larynx (EEL) is most commonly performed by Ear, Nose and Throat physicians via nasendoscopy, rigid laryngoscopy, or stroboscopy.

Nasendoscopy uses a flexible tube with a camera on the inserted end to slide through the nasal space, and down the pharynx to view the vocal folds. Rigid laryngoscopy, as the name suggests, uses a rigid column with camera, running along the tongue and then angled for a view of the vocal folds. Some clients gag with this method of assessment but experienced practitioners are often able to avoid triggering this. Videostroboscopy uses light pulses so the vocal folds look like they are moving more slowly than they are. With averages of 100 vibrations a second of the vocal folds for men and 200 for women, and an even greater number as pitch rises (Sapienza & Hoffman, 2022), it can be very helpful to see the vocal folds in "slow mo".

Some SLTs will perform their own EEL as triage or ongoing client monitoring with support from ENT colleagues whilst others will work with ENT colleagues in a joint Voice Clinic. Positively, improved therapy attendance has been noted where clients have been assessed in a multi-disciplinary clinic (Vamosi et al., 2021) and when there is not a long wait between ENT referral and voice therapy (Portone-Maira et al., 2011; Gustin et al., 2020). Interestingly, Vamosi et al. (2021) found it was the presence of an SLT which seemed to encourage onward attendance at voice therapy and Slavych et al. (2021) propose that their model of same-day ENT and SLP referral with evaluation also improves onward commitment to therapy. Our presence matters! A close and amicable relationship with ENT colleagues will also support your requests for ENT review of your clients and fosters reciprocal learning – remember you know more about the specifics of voice therapy than junior doctors!

If you are a student, ask your supervising clinician if it's possible to attend a voice-focused ENT clinic during placement, and the same applies if you are fully qualified but taking early steps in to voicework.

General practitioners

In the UK, general practitioners (GPs) are responsible for coordinating our community healthcare and will be the most likely source of referral for ENT assessment in publicly funded services. As such, any SLT reports directed to our ENT colleagues will also be copied to the client's GP. Without a medical qualification or prescribing rights, we are not able to recommend any particular medication but we can highlight areas of concern which would benefit from medical attention. This includes alerting GPs to symptoms of reflux revealed by the Reflux Symptom Index (Belafsky et al., 2002) or the Reflux Symptom Score (Lechien et al., 2020) though PPIs should not be prescribed without visualisation of the larynx (Stachler et al., 2018). They are, however, a common response to client report of throat complaints despite unconvincing evidence for their use with generalised throat symptoms (O'Hara et al., 2021) and systematic reviews regarding their use containing bias (Cosway et al., 2021).

GPs have a full record of your clients' medication and it is worth knowing common medication types including blood thinners, diuretics (or "water tablets"), anti-depressants, beta-blockers, PPIs, and inhalers to inform you about ongoing health conditions. Some medication may have an impact on the voice, such as the drying effect of antihistamines and decongestants (Stachler et al., 2018) and for UK practitioners, the online British National Formulary provides information on every drug including its purpose and side effects. You should access this if you are unfamiliar with a medication your client mentions, particularly as not all clients will be able to tell you why they take their tablets.

Respiratory physicians

Our work with upper airway disorders brings us closer to respiratory colleagues. As our involvement with this group is expanded I foresee a greater number of specialist, multidisciplinary clinics emerging in the future.

Physiotherapists

As with medical respiratory colleagues, upper airway disorders connect us to respiratory physiotherapists who will also strive for cough reduction and emergency management of UAD symptoms. Some clients will attend physiotherapy for mobility and postural issues and as we know the body can influence the voice, liaison or joint consultation with physiotherapy colleagues is valuable.

ADDITIONAL LEARNING RESOURCE

British National Formulary (online) – https://bnf.nice.org.uk/

TIP 47 – SUPPORT FOR ... MENTAL HEALTH

The influence of stress on the voice has appeared in multiple tips thus far, so I hope you've taken on board the importance of responding to this in voicework. In addition to active listening skills (Tip 7), educating clients about the link between distress and overall well-being (Tip 21) and using mindful breathing to manage their stress (Tip 22), some clients will benefit from direct support from a professional who is trained in mental health difficulties or disorders. With different support services addressing mental health from different perspectives, how do you know as a voice newbie which one to choose? Let's consider the role of each.

Psychiatry

Psychiatrists are medical professionals who have chosen to specialise in mental health disorders, in the same way, ENT colleagues chose their specialism of ears, noses, and throats. They diagnose, prescribe medication, and don't attempt to explore the client's issues. Some clients will already be known to psychiatric services with regular contact with a community psychiatric nurse (CPN), and GPs are responsible for making any new psychiatric referrals.

Psychology

Clinical psychologists adopt a problem-solving approach to mental health difficulties including cognitive behavioural therapy to break a repetitive cycle of negative thinking or reduce anxiety. A psychologist is not medically trained and cannot prescribe medications. Compared with counselling there is less focus on deep exploration of the client's issues and a greater focus on finding a solution.

Counselling

As with psychologists, counsellors are unable to prescribe medication. Instead they explore client concerns, feelings, and thoughts with an aim of clients better understanding themselves and others. There is a de-emphasis on providing advice and fixing a problem which is underpinned by the theoretical stance that the client knows themselves best and, with support, can be empowered to find their own way forward with life challenges.

TIP 48 – SUPPORT FOR ... SMOKING CESSATION

Some Health Boards or Health Trusts have a dedicated team to support anyone who wants to stop smoking and you should find out what service is available for your clients. Based within acute services and providing outreach support or located in the community, ideally we will have a direct referral route to the service. These teams may also have links with local pharmacies which provide anti-smoking medication such as nicotine patches and a "check-in" service whereby clients can discuss with the pharmacist how they're managing to reduce their cigarette consumption.

Although the most publicly recognised consequence of smoking is probably lung cancer, you know from Tip 30 (Reinke's oedema) that it can also have a significant negative impact on the voice. As an irritant, it can lead to coughing and a sensation of dryness – in fact, considering all the symptoms that can arise from smoking (even where those are not life-limiting), there is no long-term health benefit to smoking at all. Our colleagues in ENT may already have advised clients to stop smoking but as medical consultations are typically much shorter than SLT appointments, the importance of this message does not always register. We are well placed to reinforce this advice and provide voice education about why smoking should be avoided, whether clients have a specific diagnosis of Reinke's oedema or not.

In addition to a dedicated smoking cessation team in your Health Board, you can direct clients to online information, and links for the UK and Ireland are below. There is much overlap in the information provided, including reasons to stop smoking and strategies for how to do this. I would recommend you familiarise yourself with the information for your country so you can summarise what's available before recommending clients go to the website themselves.

UK AND IRELAND SMOKING CESSATION LINKS

Scotland – www.nhsinform.scot/healthy-living/stopping-smoking
England – www.nhs.uk/live-well/quit-smoking/nhs-stop-smoking-services-help-you-quit/
Wales – www.helpmequit.wales/
Northern Ireland – www.stopsmokingni.info/
Republic of Ireland – www2.hse.ie/quit-smoking/

TIP 49 – SUPPORT FOR ... EMPLOYMENT

Employers are legally required to make reasonable adjustments where workers have a physical condition, mental condition, or disability that makes their job more difficult so they are still able to carry out the duties of their job. Without reasonable adjustments, clients may need a period of sick leave which is disruptive for both employee and employer, and may attract a cost if replacement staff are required.

In England, Scotland, and Wales, employment support is provided by Access to Work, and in Northern Ireland by Access to Work (NI). Web links to the different services are provided at the end of this tip. Support from the Access to Work website includes the provision of special equipment and for our clients this could include a roaming microphone and speaker for anyone regularly projecting their voice above background noise. Outside of support provided by Access to Work, employers may consider providing support staff (Tip 41) to reduce vocal load or altering a rota to schedule a client to work during the hours with the least vocal demand. For a client working in a café this might be working at the end of the day when custom is quietening down but for a client working in a bar this might be an early shift before custom gets going. Other vocation-specific suggestions are provided in Chapter 7. Where voice difficulties are likely to be chronic (in the case of a vocal fold palsy for instance) or where there may be recurrent issues (in the case of laryngeal papillomas needing repeated surgery), changes to working patterns may need to be permanent or sufficiently flexible to accommodate repeated dysphonia.

Although many of our clients have a voice, albeit a dysphonic one, and may not appear to need someone speaking on their behalf, we do still have an advocacy role. Tips 41 and 42 touched on this with regards to us writing letters of support to GPs or employers with regards to sick leave or work adaptations. My usual approach to such correspondence is to acknowledge the commitment to voice rehab already being made by the client as a way of highlighting the shared responsibility for voice care and to show that my client is upholding their side of the bargain. This is an occupational recommendation and not just an employee hankering after upgraded furniture!

ADDITIONAL LEARNING RESOURCES

Access to Work (England, Scotland, & Wales) – www.gov.uk/access-to-work

Access to Work (NI) – www.nidirect.gov.uk/information-and-services/employment-support-people-disabilities-or-health-conditions/work-schemes-people-disabilities-or-health-conditions

TIP 50 – MULTIDISCIPLINARY WORK IN ACTION

Most clients' dysphonia is multifactorial, which often leads to multi-agency care. As you gather your case information, think about what issues are within the scope of the SLT's role and what are reliant on input from other professionals. If you can tease out what is, and isn't, your responsibility, it makes for clearer therapy planning. Outlining the different roles of the multidisciplinary team can also help clients understand their overall care plan and their part in effecting change. From everything you've picked up from the rest of the book and any clinical experience you've already had, can you think what role each of the professionals would have with the clients below? Suggested answers are in the online self-development activities.

> ### SELF-DEVELOPMENT ACTIVITY 23 – WHO SORTS WHAT?
>
> #### CLIENT 1
>
> 21-year-old female musical theatre student. Diagnosed with vocal fold nodules at ENT assessment. Uses a steroid inhaler daily for asthma which is effective in keeping symptoms under control. Has a singing teacher.
>
> - What are the SLT's responsibilities?
> - What are the ENT consultant's responsibilities?
> - What are the GP's responsibilities?
> - What are the client's responsibilities?
> - What are the singing teacher's responsibilities?
>
> #### CLIENT 2
>
> 65-year-old retired male with mild hoarseness. Diagnosed with granuloma following intubation during hospital admission for severe COVID symptoms.

- What are the SLT's responsibilities?
- What are the ENT consultant's responsibilities?
- What are the GP's responsibilities?
- What are the client's responsibilities?

Client 3

30-year-old female who works in a contact centre. Diagnosed with laryngeal papillomas. Recently had a sudden parental bereavement and is now attending a local counselling service.

- What are the SLT's responsibilities?
- What are the ENT consultant's responsibilities?
- What are the GP's responsibilities?
- What are the client's responsibilities?
- What are the counsellor's responsibilities?

REFERENCES

Belafsky, P. C., Postma, G. M. & Koufman, J. A. (2002) Validity and Reliability of the Reflux Symptom Index (RSI) *Journal of Voice* 16 (2) 274–277 https://doi.org/10.1016/s0892-1997(02)00097-8

Cosway, B., Wilson, J. A. & O'Hara, J. (2021) The Acid Test: Proton Pump Inhibitors in Persistent Throat Symptoms: A Systematic Review of Systematic Reviews. *Clinical Otolaryngology* 46 1263–1272 http://doi.org/10.1111/coa.13827

Gustin, R. L., Pielage, K. C., Howell, R., Khosla, S. & Giliberto, J. P. (2020) Increased Interval From Initial Evaluation to Initial Voice Therapy Session is Associated With Missed Voice Therapy Appointments. *Journal of Voice* 34 (6) 870–873 https://doi.org.10.1016/j.jvoice.2019.05.007

Lechien, J. R., Bobin, F., Muls, V., Thill, M-P., Horoi, M., Ostermann, K., Huet, K., Harmegnies, B., Dequanter, D.,

Dapri, G., Maréchal, M-T., Finck, C., Rodriguez Ruiz, A. & Saussez, S. (2020) Validity and Reliability of the Reflux Symptom Score. *The Laryngoscope 130* e09-e107 https://doi.org/10.1002/lary.28017

O'Hara, J., Stocken, D. D., Watson, G. C., Fouweather, T., McGlashan, J., MacKenzie, K., Carding, P., Karagama, Y., Wood, R. & Wilson, J. A (2021) Use of Proton Pump Inhibitors to Treat Persistent Throat Symptoms: Multicentre, Double Blind, Randomised, Placebo Controlled Trial. *BMJ* 372:m4903 https://doi.org/10.1136/bmj.m4903

Portone-Maira, C., Wise, J. C., Johns III, M. M. & Hapner, E. R. (2011) Differences in Temporal Variables Between Voice Therapy Completers and Dropouts. *Journal of Voice 25* (1) 62–66 https://doi.org/10.1016/j.jvoice.2009.07.007

Sapienza, C. & Hoffman, B. (2022) *Voice disorders* (4th Ed.) San Diego: Plural Publishing

Slavych, B. K., Zraick, R. I., Bursac, Z., Tulunay-Ugur, O. & Hadden, K. (2021) An Investigation of the Relationship between Adherence to Voice Therapy for Muscle Tension Dysphonia and Employment, Social Support, and Life Satisfaction. *Journal of Voice 35* (3) 386–393 https://doi.org/10.1016/j.jvoice.2019.10.015

Stachler, R. J., Francis, D. O., Schwartz, S. R., Damask, C. C., Digoy, G. P., Krouse, H. J., McCoy, S. J., Ouellette, D. R., Patel, R. R., Reavis, C. W., Smith, L. J., Smith, M., Strode, S. W., Woo, P. & Nnacheta, L. C. (2018) Clinical Practice Guideline: Hoarseness (Dysphonia) (Update). *Otolaryngology-Head and Neck Surgery (158)* (1_suppl) S1-S42 https://doi.org/10.1177/0194599817751030

Vamosi, B. E., Mikhail, L., Gustin, R. L., Pielage, K. C., Reid, K., Tabangin, M. E., Altaye, M., Collar, R. M., Khosla, S. M. Giliberto, J. P. & Howell, R. J. (2021) Predicting No Show in Voice therapy: Avoiding the Missed Appointment Cycle. *Journal of Voice 35* (4) 604–608 https://doi.org/10.1016/j.jvoice.2020.01.003

Chapter 9

LEARNING FROM CLIENTS

So far, research evidence has been provided with each clinically relevant tip to support its rationale but what happens when we apply our knowledge to real people?

This chapter presents three client accounts, written by former clients themselves, which include both the challenges and successes of therapy. Each story can be read individually, although there are some common threads across the accounts. Amanda Lynne's, Rory's, and Eliza Kath's experiences of voice therapy bring together many of the different tips and by the end of this chapter you should have a sense of therapy in action and appreciate the meaningfulness of SLT input for voice difficulties. Enjoy!

LEARN FROM ... AMANDA LYNNE

Diagnosis: vocal fold nodules with secondary muscle tension dysphonia and concomitant reflux

I am a musician, singer, instrumental teacher and workshop leader and have successfully overcome voice difficulties with speech and language therapy.

Four years ago I kept feeling my throat was dry and sore, and would lose my voice quite a bit. I was diagnosed with pre-nodules at an ENT consultation which had developed through overuse from singing, lots of teaching, socialising, and laughing, and misuse from being too loud and using my breath incorrectly. I also had pretty bad acid reflux.

I had a course of speech therapy to avoid doing any more damage and was given a couple of exercises to do – mostly sentences to try to get better control of my breath. I have to admit, I didn't fully engage with this round of treatment, and there were a few factors that led me to take it less seriously. My voice felt hoarse and a bit sore but I could still force out a song and chat, so I wasn't as worried. I felt a bit embarrassed saying I was a musician as didn't want the therapist to think I was lying but I didn't connect with the therapy. I didn't really feel any difference after doing the exercises, and some of the handouts went straight over my head. I couldn't always connect the printouts to what I was feeling and didn't really understand the aim. I wasn't prepared with questions and I didn't get into a daily routine of implementing the exercises, so didn't see a positive outcome. That's my responsibility, although I think I needed a slightly more tailored approach due to the varied nature of my work. It did make me a bit more aware though, and I spent a few months being careful. I used a steam inhaler most days, and got a bit better at my mic technique but it didn't take long to make the silly mistake of slipping back into old habits and my days were as full as ever of voice-demanding activities.

A couple of years later was one of my busiest voice years ever. When I wasn't away performing or teaching, I'd play local pub gigs, and if I wasn't doing that I'd catch up with friends in the pub and play tunes, shout about, laugh, and sing songs. I'm a very sociable person! With every summer gig there were friends to catch up with, post-gig socialising, and lots and lots of long drives where we spent hours blethering. Unfortunately that led to fully developed nodules although these were soft so still reversible. I went back to speech therapy with a different therapist and was instantly advised to have a month of vocal rest with no singing or teaching, and speaking was limited in its amount and to a lower volume in quiet environments. I also needed to make a conscious effort to remove acid-creating stuff from my diet. One coffee a week was my limit, and I still stick to limited caffeine and plenty of water now. I stopped boozing too, as that only created more acid and meant I also forgot to be quiet. I managed to avoid singing and shouting but had to have some quiet chatting to avoid losing my head. Notebooks became my replacement voice for the majority of the time.

My voice soon started to change with the voice rest so the next challenge was re-learning how to use it in different situations which would stop the nodules from returning if we could get rid of them. There would be exercises to help me get rid of the tension in my throat and larynx too. I took the exercises seriously this time, and we worked to create a program that I could clearly understand the reasoning behind.

I learned that I don't only need to warm up for gigs, but for teaching large or loud workshops too as I have to shout. The teaching is actually more straining sometimes and online teaching can be a killer. Each day in the shower I focus on exercises to warm up my conversational voice making sure my throat feels wide, I can say individual sounds, words, and sentences, I can vary the notes, and finally I vary the volume using a quiet, medium, and loud voice. For a full warm-up before a gig or workshop I use similar exercises but also massage my neck, throat, jaw, and cheeks with a focus on losing any tension. When I vary my projection and pitch I try to cover the full range I'll be using in a gig. If a note is missing or hoarse during my warm-up I'll use sirening as a gentle way to stretch my range.

I knew I'd done damage to my voice the second time round as I could feel it and suddenly got worried I was jeopardising my career. I really regretted not doing it properly the first time as I came really close to having to give up my profession. I got a bit of a telling off at the ENT appointment and although I felt a bit annoyed about that at the time, it scared me into taking the vocal rest seriously and when the therapy started I was desperate to see if I could get my voice back. That want to improve, teamed with a therapist who took time to look at how I actually used and needed my voice, made it feel positive. I understood why I was doing each thing, and didn't feel bombarded with handouts. Bite-sized pieces really helped and I didn't feel rushed. Having a structured routine which gets added to every session felt manageable. I needed exercises that suit different environments (I don't always get a dressing room!) and the therapist and I worked on creating a plan together which I still use when on tour.

Although it took a while to get to grips with actually understanding what certain body feelings meant, therapy taught me to be self-aware and it's so important to listen to your body. If your voice hurts don't use it. Being self-employed, I find it hard to turn down any work, but if there isn't a night off in 2 months then you need to factor in some down time and not feel bad about it. It might be the recovery time your voice needs to keep going! Before it was explained to me, I think I was really ignorant to how my voice actually worked and how I'd done the damage and because of that it took me a while to get the exercises right. I had to persevere a bit and make sure I prepared questions for appointments if there was anything I couldn't do right. I remember when I first felt my throat widen properly rather than clenching my tongue and it was like a light bulb going off. I'd never been aware of that feeling before. It was really helpful to check sensations with my fingers on my neck and I still do that.

LEARN FROM ... RORY

Diagnosis: primary muscle tension dysphonia with subsequent diagnosis of reflux

There were a number of things on our first call that really helped me. First, it was the broad diagnosis – as always, it's nice to be told "this doesn't sound like a serious physical injury". It immediately helped me to engage with what came next and I wasn't half in my mind thinking "great, but I need to see that ENT specialist to get scoped…" Knowing something can be fixed without surgery motivates the desire to then DO WHAT YOU'RE TOLD… [client's own capitals]

The next immediate thing that was very helpful was the deconstriction exercises. They definitely worked, but I will never know how much it was the physical practice of doing the exercise, the psychosomatic factor of believing in the process and thus relaxing, or simply the practice of not worrying every time I made a noise. But it definitely worked physically and that (again, obviously in my case) was an important "anchor" for the rest – I knew there were practical things I could do and that they had an effect.

So in summary, (a) I believed it could be fixed and (b) early interventions worked for me and that motivated me to do them. Those were both important. From there, for me, by far the most important things were understanding how my vocal system worked and understanding a few techniques to help me assess and understand what was happening. So I think in roughly chronological order:

The explanation of constriction was very important. Even more so, the metaphor you used of an ankle injury and "relearning" how to do something you already knew how to do was crucial for me. That one analogy did more than almost any single thing. I UNDERSTOOD what I'd done and even recognised the how and why of what I'd done. I could feel myself doing it because I understood it in that analogy. It may be that the fact I had experience of the other half of the analogy (ankle injuries and changed gait) helped but either way, the understanding of the process was very important.

Likewise I can't overstate how important the idea of "me pushing sound using muscles high up rather than pushing sound with my chest and shaping it" was to seeing what was going on. I thought about that a lot – so much so I can't actually remember how you phrased it because I kind of rephrased that in my head to understand it my way. I don't THINK I distorted the meaning but it was important.

The weird exercise you had me do with opening my mouth wide while doing an ungainly downwards smile was also something that was good for me. Not only was this the deconstriction technique which worked best for me, it helped me physically understand the shape of my throat and what it was doing. If the two points above helped me understand what was going on, this one helped me feel it.

Also, the example you gave of primary school teachers raising their pitch to sound friendly and engaging was very useful for me because I do it a lot. In fact, I'm still battling that one all the time because I do it reflexively whenever I get passionate or excited in a conversation (which is quite a lot).

I've had other experiences of voice therapy which have been mixed. My previous speech therapist nearly lost me during my first phone consultation and first in-person session because she started from a very low base with some very basic breathing exercises which I already knew well. She won me over later but she HAD to win me over because I was virtually saying out loud "look, I realise you get a lot of patients with no background in having even tried mindfulness or stretching or relaxation and breathing techniques but you already know I have because we talked about it…". That said, she explained how my breathing physically worked, which was helpful. People keep talking about the diaphragm going up and down when you breathe. No-one had every explained to me that it goes in the opposite direction to what it feels like it does. I assumed that as you breath "up" and your lungs fill up, your diaphragm was going up. It meant that when focusing on my breathing I tended to make my stomach do the opposite of what it should have been – pulling it "in and up" to fill up my lungs. It made a substantial difference to actually understand how my breathing worked. Again, that didn't have immediate practical implications exactly but it helped me understand what was going on and why and helped me to find my own ways to do things better.

Later she gave me a kind of "resonant frequency" exercise which helped me to understand better where my natural pitch was. That REALLY helped because I realised I was way more comfortable at a lower speaking pitch than I was used to. I had theorised this myself; one night I was supposed to be having dinner with friends and nearly didn't go because I'd talked a lot that week and my voice was really tired and throat a bit sore. I decided to go but was very sensitive about being deliberate about talking and how. I sat up very straight and thought about breathing from my chest. I realised later that it had caused me to speak in a deeper tone and not only did it let me get through the night, it actually left me feeling better than I'd started. I talked quite a bit that night and it got better, not worse. I asked about this, got the exercise which I adapted myself to do a nasal hum that starts low in pitch and rise to high at pitch. I put a hand on my chest and my nose and I can become aware the point at which chest vibration starts to be replaced with nasal vibration and it helped me visualise where my natural range was. This is my ongoing biggest challenge – talk at my own pitch.

Another thing that that all involved was understanding the lining of the throat and irritation. At first I dismissed the whole acid reflux thing because I don't get a lot of heartburn and I had preconceived ideas about who gets reflux but when it was properly explained to me I immediately went "eh, no, wait a minute, I get that quite a bit don't I?" The ENT specialist put me back on omeprazole for a couple of months and yes, it makes a difference. This is, I think, what is new about all this – I realise my separate-but-happened-at-the-same-time stomach issues weren't separate at all and are probably behind the fairly recent phenomena of extra acid reflux. Again, simply understanding helped me to recognise what was happening and that also made a difference.

Essentially, when I have the right combination of "belief it can be better", "evidence it can be better", "real, proper understanding of what is wrong and why", and "some basic tools to help me fix it", I'm generally good to go, committed and motivated and I think about it a lot (too much, I know). Others may be way more practically minded than me and benefit from repetition and guidelines. I have a sheet of paper with exercises but I only do a fraction of them because I feel and understand what works for me. Others may do better just systematically working through a programme. I'm bad with being patient with steps I don't feel work or where I can see them "fixing" one of the things that wasn't really wrong for me.

Person-centred medicine strongly applies to where a patient starts from physically and psychologically. Understanding people is about more than just a diagnosis. And understanding people is really helpful in getting them to do stuff. That was what I found wrong with a physio session years ago – I had 15 minutes to be given exercises I had done before because the physio had a six-week backlog and no time for some inquisitive rugby player asking her a raft of questions. I am empathetic – but it didn't work…

LEARN FROM … ELIZA KATH

Diagnosis: muscle tension dysphonia of no obvious origin

Voice therapists definitely need to look at the body as well as listening to the voice as I didn't realise I was holding so much tension until it was pointed out to me. Fledgling therapists definitely need to understand that not everything is a quick fix and that patience is required since improvement doesn't come overnight, especially if it's been a long-term issue. In fact I think as we get older nothing is a quick fix and not everything actually ever gets completely fixed. I'm thinking of other body injuries which we can work with until they get to a point that they are manageable and I guess the same is with the voice, although I never seem to find the thing that works to keep it manageable. I feel as though I'm destined to always have struggles with my voice and it pains me to say that.

SELF-DEVELOPMENT ACTIVITY **24** – REFLECTION ON LEARNING FROM CLIENTS

Now that you have read these genuine accounts of clients' experiences of voice therapy, what will you take into your practice? There are no right or wrong answers here!

PUBLISHED ASSESSMENTS

SINGING VOICE HANDICAP INDEX-10 (COHEN ET AL., 2009)

Instructions: These are statements that many people have used to describe their singing and the effects of their singing on their lives. Circle the response that indicates how frequently you have had the same experience in the last four weeks.

Appendix 1: Published Assessments

		0 = Never	1 = Almost Never	2 = Sometimes	3 = Almost Always	4 = Always
1.	It takes a lot of effort to sing	0	1	2	3	4
2.	I am unsure of what will come out when I sing	0	1	2	3	4
3.	My voice "gives out" on me while I am singing	0	1	2	3	4
4.	My singing voice upsets me		1	2	3	4
5.	I have no confidence in my singing voice	0	1	2	3	4
6.	I have trouble making my voice do what I want it to	0	1	2	3	4
7.	I have to "push it" to produce my voice when singing	0	1	2	3	4
8.	My singing voice tires easily	0	1	2	3	4
9.	I feel something is missing in my life because of my inability to sing	0	1	2	3	4
10.	I am unable to use my "high voice"	0	1	2	3	4

VOICE TRACT DISCOMFORT SCALE (VTDS) (MATHIESON ET AL., 2009)

The following are symptoms or sensations that you may feel in your throat, which may occur as part of your voice problem. Please indicate the **frequency** with which they occur and the **severity** of the symptom/sensation, by circling a number in the appropriate column.

Patient identifier:	Frequency of sensation/symptom							Severity of sensation/symptom						
Date:	Never	sometimes		often		always		none		mild		moderate		extreme
	0	1	2	3	4	5	6	0	1	2	3	4	5	6
1 Burning	0	1	2	3	4	5	6	0	1	2	3	4	5	6
2 Tightness	0	1	2	3	4	5	6	0	1	2	3	4	5	6
3 Dry	0	1	2	3	4	5	6	0	1	2	3	4	5	6
4 Aching	0	1	2	3	4	5	6	0	1	2	3	4	5	6
5 Tickling	0	1	2	3	4	5	6	0	1	2	3	4	5	6
6 Sore	0	1	2	3	4	5	6	0	1	2	3	4	5	6
7 Irritable	0	1	2	3	4	5	6	0	1	2	3	4	5	6
8 Lump in the throat	0	1	2	3	4	5	6	0	1	2	3	4	5	6

THERAPY RESOURCES

WHAT IS CONTRIBUTING TO MY VOICE DIFFICULTIES?

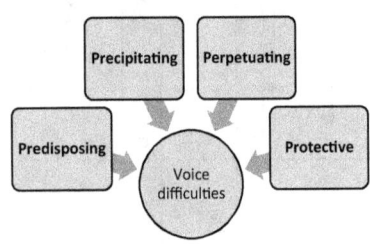

- Predisposing – what increases my risk of having voice problems?
- Precipitating – what has caused this episode of voice difficulties?
- Perpetuating – what is keeping the voice difficulties going?
- Protective – what can help me reduce the voice difficulties or my risk of voice difficulties?

	Predisposing	Precipitating	Perpetuating	Protective
My physical health				
My mental health				
My environment				
My vocal care				
My voice production style				

MAXIMISING BREATH GROUPS

We need to have enough breath to support our voice in conversations because running out of air may lead to strain. Use the sentences below to identify where you can most comfortably pause to take a breath, and ensure you never run out of air. Try to practice taking regular top-up breaths when you're speaking with others.

I went for a walk (5)
I went for a walk today (7)
I went for a walk today across the fields (11)
I went for a walk today across the fields and it was sunny (16)
I went for a walk today across the fields and it was sunny and hot (18)
I went for a walk today across the fields and it was sunny and hot with a good view (22)
I went for a walk today across the fields and it was sunny and hot with a good view of the countryside (27)
I went for a walk today across the fields and it was sunny and hot with a good view of the countryside so I rested on a rock (34)
I went for a walk today across the fields and it was sunny and hot with a good view of the countryside so I rested on a rock and drank some water (39)
I went for a walk today across the fields and it was sunny and hot with a good view of the countryside so I rested on a rock and drank some cool and refreshing water (44)

USEFUL RESOURCES

With so many sources of information in this book, I have distilled the key resources and would recommend you look up these resources to start you on your way.

Brassett, C., Evans, E. & Fay, I. (2017) *The Secret Language of Anatomy. An Illustrated Guide to the Origins of Anatomical Terms.* Chichester: Anatomy Boutique Books

Dimon, T. (2018) *Anatomy of the Voice. An Illustrated Guide for Singers, Vocal Coaches, and Speech Therapists.* Berkeley: North Atlantic Books

Martin, S. (2021) *Working With Voice Disorders. Theory and Practice.* (3rd Ed.) Abingdon: Routledge

Sapienza, C. & Hoffman, B. (2022) *Voice disorders* (4th Ed.) San Diego: Plural Publishing

Shewell, C. (2009) *Voice Work. Art and Science in Changing Voices.* Chichester: Wiley-Blackwell

ADDITIONAL LEARNING RESOURCES

Voice Science Works – a website distilling contemporary research for use by any voice user. It has useful downloadable resources and educational videos. www.voicescienceworks.org/

SUGGESTED INSTAGRAM ACCOUNTS TO FOLLOW

@voicefituk – a UK specialist voice therapist, Tor Spence, runs this account. She has a particular interest in chronic cough and upper airway disorders

@voicecarecentre – a London voice centre specialising in vocal manual therapy. Their multidisciplinary team includes

SLTs, a vocal rehab coach, an Osteopath, a Mindset Coach and Nutritional Scientist

@vocologyireland – a singing teacher, Eimar McCarthy Luddy, runs this account. She has an interest in vocal health for singing and loves her anatomy with fun quizzes and helpful diagrams to help the layperson understand the layout of the vocal tract

@kristie_voice – this is Kirstie Knickerbocker's account and I cite some of her work in this text. She is an American speech and language therapist and voice specialist

INDEX

Abraham, C. 24
Access to Work 89, 179, 206, 207
adherence 27
Adler, R. K 6
agency 29, 30
Aghadoost, S. 128
Aiken, P. J. 175, 190
Allison, L. H. 71, 191
Alves, I. A. V. 175
Alves, M. 91
Alwani, M. M. 40
Assad, J. P. 70, 132, 176
assessment: acoustic 45, 46, 65, 66, 158, 185; Cough Severity Index 148; endoscopic 64, 129, 143, 199; perceptual 18, 46, 65–66, 158, 185; Reflux Symptom Index 200; Reflux Symptom Score 200; Singing Voice Handicap Index 185; Voice Handicap Index 67, 185
asthma 76, 77, 94, 123, 148, 208
atrophy 48, 151, 152
awareness: 93, 96, 98–101, 102–103, 117, 128, 132, 173, 180

background noise 3, 15, 37, 69, 153, 174, 176, 183, 190, 206
Baker, J. 129, 130, 131
Ballestas, S. A. 160
Bastian, R. W. 69, 132
Behlau, M. 28, 29, 134

Behrman, A. 67
Belafsky, M. A. 153, 200
botulinum toxin 154, 155
Brassett, C. 5
breathing 42; in generalisation 114, 115; meditation 107–108, 202; mouth 92–93; nasal 92; phrasing 105–107, 180; placement 105; relaxation 107; spaces 96, 99–100; surgery 146; upper airway disorders 149
British Association for Performing Arts Medicine (BAPAM) 188, 189, 192
British Voice Association (BVA) 91
Burleson, B. R. 24, 53
Burns, K. 28
Büyükatalay, Z. C. 56

caffeine 15, 92, 141, 213
Cantarella, G. 71, 182
CAPE-V scale *see* assessment, perceptual
Cardoso, N. S. V. 109, 111
change: challenges to 51–53, 79, 138; facilitating/supporting 13, 22–26, 27–28, 29–30, 39–41, 98–101, 102, 103; outcomes 46–47, 66, 88, 148; policy 50
Chiu, J. C-H 3
chronic cough 148–149, 150

classification 74–75; new terminology 74; non-organic 74–75; organic 74–75, 123
client as own therapist 23, 48, 102
client stories 212–218
coaching questions 28, 29, 39, 134
cognitive activation 41
cognitive behavioural therapy 131, 202
Cohen, S. M. 185
collaboration 27–28, 44, 48, 56, 89, 133
compliance *see* adherence
conducting therapy: feedback 7, 31, 41, 43–45, 98, 105, 110, 111, 128; instructions 40, 52; modelling 30, 40, 51, 72, 153
confidentiality 35, 131
confidential voice 94
contributing factors 76–77
Conversation Training Therapy 115
Cook-Cunningham, S. L. 192
cool down exercises 38, 187–188, 192–193
Cosway, B. 200
counselling 32–33, 80, 130–131, 202, 209
cultural responsiveness 55–57; and Cultural Atlas 55, 56, 61
cysts 164

de Almeida, R. B. S. 146
de Brito Mota, A. F. 176
decision making: discharge 32, 41, 45, 48, 54, 78–80; planning therapy 76, 87–89, 104, 208
deconstruction exercises *see* direct therapy
Dehqan, A. 123, 128
Dejonckere, P. H 65, 72

Desjardins, M. 152, 153
Dimon, T. 5
direct therapy: deconstruction exercises 127, 128, 192, 215, 216; semi-occluded vocal tract exercises 109–113; strengthening exercises 143, 146
Doll, E. J. 36
Doruk, C. 40
Dueppen, A. J. 40

Eastwood, C. 39
Ebersole, B. 27, 29, 67, 87, 151, 173
employment *see* work
Enderby, P. 46
Estes, C. 175, 190
evidence-based practice 27, 40, 42, 47, 52
Evitts, P. M. 3
experimentation: in assessment 72–73; client 57, 112, 157; reader 16–17, 22

Faham, M. 155
feedback *see* conducting therapy
Flynn, A. 175
functional voice disorder 123–128

Gartner-Schmidt, J. 115, 116
generalisation *see* transfer of skills
Georgalas, V. L. 91
Gillespie, A. 46, 48, 132
Gottliebson, A. 15
granulomas 141–142, 147, 208
GRBAS scale *see* assessment, perceptual
Gray, H. 131

Greve, K. 175
Grillo, E. U. 175
Gustin, R. L. 199

Hacki, T. 74, 123
Halvorsen, T. 149
Hassan, E. M. 65
hearing loss 153
Heppner, W. L. 97
Hintze, J. 154
Hogikyan, N. D. 67
home practice 45, 53, 57, 106
Hughes, S. M. 3
Hunter, E. J. 69
Hutchins, S. D. 164
hydration: nebulisation 56, 91, 92, 94; steam inhalations 15, 17, 56, 91, 92, 94, 193, 212; water 15, 38, 76, 77, 91–92, 94, 213

impact: assessment 63–67; emotional 87; functional 87; occupational 89; of posture 15, 37; stress 100, 130; of therapy 49–50; of voice difficulties 2–3, 80, 87, 88, 90, 148, 155; indirect therapy 91–95; for specific diagnoses 127, 129, 138, 141, 143, 151, 154, 160, 163, 164
inducible laryngeal obstruction 46, 149–150
Instagram accounts 11, 227
Ishikawa, K. 3
Iwarsson, J.: breathing 104, 105; conducting therapy 41, 98; negative practice 42, 99; student development 5; transfer of skills 114, 115, 116

Jacobsen, B. H. 67, 185
Jannetts, S. 66

Jo, Y. 133
Joseph, B. E. 15
Joshi, A. 157

Kabat-Zinn, J. 99
Kaneko, M. 109, 157
Kang, C. H. 128
Kenny, C. 36
Khodeir, M. S. 139
Kishbaugh, K. C. 36
Knickerbocker, K. 15, 38, 164
Korn, G. P. 3, 174
Kuhlmann, L. L. 106

laryngeal cysts *see* cysts
laryngeal papillomas *see* papillomas
laryngeal polyps *see* polyps
Lechien, J. R. 200
Lee, Y. S. 163
Leeuw, M. 126
Lyberg-Åhlander, V. 3

Madill, C. 39, 40, 87, 102, 120, 123, 127
Mannix, K. 27, 32
Mansouri, Y. 3
manual therapy 11, 37, 97, 128, 188, 227
Marques Torbes, T. M. 27
Martin, S. 5, 63, 87, 90, 91, 99, 176, 192
Martins, R. H. G. 140
Mathieson, L. 5, 67
medical: assessment 141, 148, 204; liaison 200; management 154; problems 47, 53, 63, 92, 123; *see also* asthma; reflux
medication 53, 94, 141, 148, 200, 202, 204; and British National Formulary 200, 201

Medina, A. M. 96, 98, 99–100
meditation 4, 81, 96–97, 99–100, 104, 107–108
Meier, B. 175
mental health 33–34, 35, 77, 188, 202–203
mentoring *see* supervision
Meyer, T. K. 155
Mills, R. D. 109
mind-body connection 63, 96–97
mindfulness *see* meditation
mirening *see* sirening
modelling 30, 40, 51, 72, 153
Morrow, S. L. 71
multidisciplinary working: counselling 32–33, 80, 130–131, 202–203, 209; Ear, Nose and Throat consultant 199–200; general practitioner 200; physiotherapy 201; psychiatry 202; psychology 202; respiratory physician 80, 148, 200–201
muscle tension dysphagia 128
muscle tension dysphonia: primary 53, 123, 129, 214, 218; secondary 103, 126, 139, 162, 164

Nakagawa, H. 163
Naunheim, M. R. 3
negative practice 42, 99, 110, 111
nodules 48, 74, 91, 103, 104, 132–137, 181, 208, 212

Öcal, B. 163
O'Hara, J. 200
onward referral 79, 80, 97, 131
outcomes 46–50; and optimising 27, 39, 89, 157, 173

palsies 74, 143–147
papillomas 4, 46, 88, 103, 126, 158, 160–162, 163, 206, 209
Park, J. H. 153
Parker, L. A. 161
Petrizzo, D. 66
physical health 76– 77 199–201
planning therapy *see* decision making
polyps 137, 163
Pomaville, F. 175
Porcaro, C. K. 3, 175
Portone-Maira, C. 199
posture 15, 30, 36, 37, 126, 174, 175, 179, 182
presbycusis *see* hearing loss
presbyphonia 48, 64, 151–153
professional voice users: airline workers 174; contact centre workers 182–184, 209; educators 175, 176–181; fitness instructors 190–191; health professionals 175; performers 173, 185–189; taxi drivers 173, 174; tour guides 173, 174–175
progress: facilitating factors 29, 39; hindering factors 43; slower 23, 51–54, 138, 153
projection 71, 72, 135, 153, 158, 180, 213
psychogenic voice disorder 75, 90, 129–131

reflux 54, 92, 141, 142, 149, 163, 200, 212, 214
Reinke's oedema 64, 81, 127, 138–140, 204
relaxation 104, 107, 135, 216
remote therapy 36–38, 61, 76
Renk, E. 185

Rihkanen, H. 157, 158
Roddam, H. 52
Rohlfing, M. L. 3
Rosen, C. A. 67, 185
Royal College of Speech and Language Therapists (RCSLT) 2, 36, 91, 121
Rubino, M. 27, 40
Rumbach, A. F. 4, 5, 7, 15, 18, 30, 175, 190

Sanssené, C. 174
Sapienza, C. 5, 199
Schroeder, S. R. 3
Searl, J. 15
self-development activities 13, 14, 16, 17, 18, 25, 31, 33, 35, 50, 55, 64, 67, 80, 100, 111, 112, 136, 146, 186, 208, 219
self-efficacy 29–31
self-regulation 29
semi-occluded vocal tract exercises *see* direct therapy
Shewell, C.: breathing 115; clinical resource 5, 90, 120; extension skills 89; performing voice 185; professional voice user groups 173; vocal tract expansion 109; Voice Skills Framework 104, 127; Voice Skills Perceptual Profile 63, 87
sick leave *see* work
singing teacher 11, 188, 208, 228
singing voice 14, 126, 136, 185–188, 192, 208, 212
sirening 186, 187, 213
Slavych, B. K. 27, 29, 199
smoking: cessation 24, 34, 81, 91, 92, 138, 204–205; harm of 4, 138–139

social cognitive therapy 24
solution-focused brief therapy 28
spasmodic dysphonia 88, 154–155
Spellman, J. 3
Stachler, R. J. 63, 154, 200
strain: as audible symptom 104, 123, 129, 138, 153, 154, 160, 163; breath-related 105–106, 180, 184, 193; on perceptual assessment 19, 65, 66; as physical symptom 87, 102, 103, 124, 146, 174
stretches 15, 97, 179, 193
Sundar, K. M. 148
supervision 5, 7, 43, 52, 57, 111, 131
surgery 137, 139–140, 143, 156–159, 160–161, 163, 206
swallowing 74, 94, 128, 143, 146
Sylvestre, A. 39

teaching: environment 70, 176–177; projection 180–181; style 177–178; support 178–179
tender conversations 32–35, 88, 130, 131, 149
tension *see* muscle tension dysphagia *and* muscle tension dysphonia
Tezcaner, Z. C. 131
therapist voice: looking after 37–38; reflection on 13–14, 15–17
throat clearing 16, 91, 93, 94, 148, 156
transfer of skills 48, 98, 114–118
Tyrmi, J. 111

upper airway disorders 148–150, 200–201

Vamosi, B. E. 199
Vanderaa, V. 154
Van Houtte, E. 3, 175, 176
van Leer, E.: adherence 27; and awareness 98; change 22; client preferences 42; practice 29, 40, 51, 115, 116; self-efficacy 30; self-management 41; social cognitive therapy 24; stress 96
Van Lierde, K. M. 15
Villar, A. 3, 174
vocal athletes 173–175
vocal dose: overdoers 69, 70, 132; underdoers 69, 71, 151
vocal fold nodules *see* nodules
vocal fold palsies *see* palsies
vocal health 78, 88, 98, 102, 127, 179, 188, 190
voice clinic 18–19, 141, 199
voice conservation 16, 34, 71, 132–133, 191
voice diaries 98–99, 136
voice education 98; and pre-operative 156; preventative 175; vocal health 98, 204

Warhurst, S. 15
warm-ups 38, 192–193; and BAPAM 97, 188–189, 197; humming 110; for presbyphonia 152; for singers 186–188, 213; semi-occluded vocal tract exercises 112; for teachers 179
White, A. C. 22, 40, 156, 158
Wilson, J. A. 3
work: environment 15, 36, 70, 76, 157, 173, 174, 176, 190; equipment 175, 179, 182–183, 190–191, 206; pattern 182; sick leave 50, 88, 158, 181, 186, 206; stress 175, 176, 182, 184; support 206–207
working collaboratively *see* collaboration

Yorkston, K. 155
Young, V. N. 151

Zenari, M. S. 109, 112, 175
Zhuge, P. 163
Ziegler, A. 151
Zraick, R. I. 66

For Product Safety Concerns and Information please contact our EU
representative GPSR@taylorandfrancis.com
Taylor & Francis Verlag GmbH, Kaufingerstraße 24, 80331 München, Germany

www.ingramcontent.com/pod-product-compliance
Lightning Source LLC
Chambersburg PA
CBHW060600230426
43670CB00011B/1909